Monographs on Endocrinology

Volume 9

Edited by

F. Gross, Heidelberg · M. M. Grumbach, San Francisco · A. Labhart, Zürich

M. B. Lipsett, Cleveland · T. Mann, Cambridge

L. T. Samuels, Salt Lake City · J. Zander, München

Monographs on Endocrinology

R.E.Mancini

Immunologic Aspects of Testicular Function

With 36 Figures

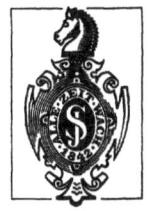

Springer-Verlag Berlin · Heidelberg · New York 1976

Prof. Dr. ROBERTO E. MANCINI
Centro de Investigationes en Reproduccion
Facultad de Medicina – 10°P. Universidad de Buenos Aires
Buenos Aires – Argentina

ISBN-13: 978-3-642-80987-3   e-ISBN-13: 978-3-642-80985-9
DOI: 10.1007/978-3-642-80985-9

Library of Congress Cataloging in Publication Data. Mancini, Roberto E. Immunologic aspects of testicular function. (Monographs on endocrinology; v. 9) Bibliography: p. 000 Includes index. 1. Testicle – Diseases – Immunological aspects. I. Title. RC898.M36 616.6′8′079 75-31730

To my wife, my daughter and my son

Contents

Introduction

It has become increasingly evident within the last few decades that immunologic factors are involved in some aspects of the reproductive process and hence in the physiology and pathology of the genital tract.

The concept that immune phenomena participate in human reproduction is not new. There are examples throughout the history of man that immune phenomena may have influenced the reproductive process. For example, the Bible states that Sarah was sterile for a long time but conceived in the later years of her marriage. This could be interpreted to mean that continued exposure to her husband's ejaculated antigens resulted in antibody response, sufficient to induce sterility. However, after continence of long duration, the antibody level declined and conception became possible. Another source of speculation is Darwin's *Descent of Man,* which contains a number of statements to the effect that profligacy of women may account for their "small fertility". The inference is that repeated exposure to antigenic material in the ejaculate causes antibody responses that lead to infertility (KATSH and KATSH, 1965). This is directly related to the modern postulate that prostitutes do not conceive because of antisperm antibodies acquired by frequent contact with semen.

Clear-cut demonstration of the antigenic power of spermatozoa or of whole semen in heterologous inoculation was first presented towards the end of the last century (LANDSTEINER, 1899; METCHNIKOFF, 1900). In an effort to develop a simple way to prevent conception, attempts were made to damage seminiferous epithelium in the male, or to inhibit fertility in the female animal, by inducing sperm antibodies. It was not until twenty years ago that investigators began to focus their attention on the problem that sperm antigens and antibodies may be pathogenically related to human male and female infertility. In the case of the male, this idea was reinforced by the emerging evidence of the existence of autoimmune disease, which causes a given tissue to behave as foreign to its own host. As a consequence it induces the development of specific autoantibodies which destroy analogous tissues or cells throughout the body. These self-perpetuating diseases have their equivalent in the reproductive male organs. The testicular tissue, sperm cells, seminal plasma, and the male accessory glands possess enough antigenic potency to induce autoantibody formation which can render the male organism temporarily or permanently sterile. These observations attracted the interest of numerous researchers and as a result a promising and fascinating area of investigation known as immunoreproduction has developed. This biological and clinical discipline is at present concerned with the elucidation of the etiology of unexplained infertility and also the possibility that early abortion, hydatid mole and choriocarcinoma may arise from immunologic impairment.

This review has been divided into three parts, each of which is dedicated to a special aspect of immunoreproduction in the male. The first part describes the experimental background in terms of antigens, antibodies, pathology, pathogenesis, and inhibition of the so-called experimental allergic or immunologic orchitis which results from the sperm antigen-antibody interaction. The second part is devoted to clinical findings which include the induction of human orchitis, the antigenicity of testis, spermatozoa, and accessory glands as revealed by the development of corresponding antibodies and tissue damage. In the third part a detailed description is given of the different anti-sperm antibodies, lesions of testis and accessory glands found in sterile patients, and the causal relationships operative in immunologic pathogenesis of male sterility are discussed.

Our primary objective has been to provide up-to-date information for biologists, immunologists, pathologists and physicians interested in immunoreproduction, together with a critical review of the possible mechanisms whereby immunologic factors affect the process of spermatogenesis.

I. Experimental Immunologic Orchitis

1. Antigenicity of Testis

Evidence of the antigenicity of testis and semen was first presented at the end of the last century. LANDSTEINER (1899), METCHNIKOFF (1900), and METALNIKOFF (1900) demonstrated the induction of a "spermotoxic" antibody in animals sensitized with testicular homogenate or semen; this antibody was capable of immobilizing sperm cells. Sera from rabbits immunized with sheep semen, immobilized rat sperm by heterologous sensitization (VON MOXTER, 1900). When rabbits were sensitized with either bovine or human testicular homogenate, the resulting immune sera showed precipitating reactions with the corresponding testis, suggesting species specificity (FARNUM, 1901; STRUBE, 1902). The repeated inoculation of chickens with rabbit sperm provoked the formation of an *in vitro* immobilizing antibody not only against rabbits but guinea

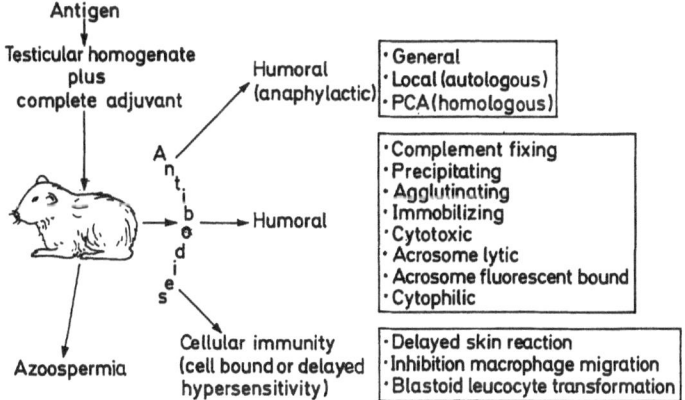

Fig. 1. A list of different types of humoral antibodies, cellular immunity, and spermatogenic response obtained after immunization of adult guinea pigs with testicular antigens mixed with complete Freund's adjuvant

pigs as well (GUYER, 1922). The earliest demonstration of a homologous type of antisperm sensitization (KENNEDY, 1924) was the immobilization of spermatozoa, and in some cases atrophy of germinal epithelium, following repeated injections of testicular homogenate or epididymal sperm. Homologous and heterologous cross reactions between testis and brain in rabbits were demonstrated for the first time by injecting animals with alcohol-extractable material from either organ; species and organ specificity was assessed by negative results obtained with liver, kidney, and lungs (LEWIS, 1934).

Real progress widening the concepts of immunologic impairment of spermatogenesis was made when a selective destruction of germinal cells was obtained in guinea pigs by auto- or homologous sensitization with a single dose of homogenate prepared from testicular tissue, semen, or spermatozoa, to which FREUND's complete adjuvant was added. The testis lesions were accompanied by development of humoral antibodies and cellular immunity (VOISIN et. al., 1951; DELAUNAY and VOISIN, 1952; FREUND et. al., 1953). The same testicular response, but of lower incidence and magnitude, could be obtained when repeated injections of testis homogenate alone were given for several months, without adjuvant (BISHOP, 1961). With the exception of a

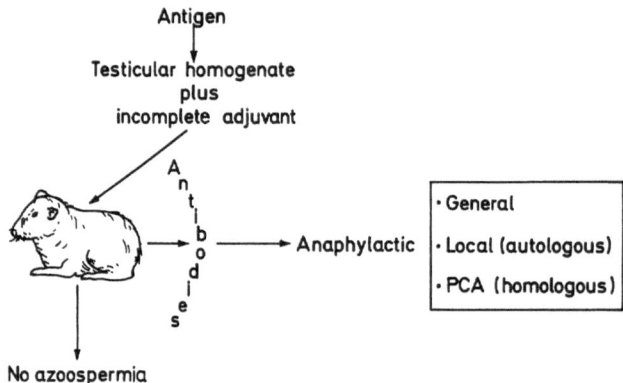

Fig. 2. Only certain types of humoral antibodies are developed by adult guinea pigs after sensitization with testicular antigens mixed with incomplete Freund's adjuvant

cross reaction with brain tissue, as already mentioned, the induced allergic or immunologic aspermatogenesis or azoospermia has a high degree of organ and species specificity. Although less susceptible than the guinea pigs, other species such as adult mice (POKORNA et al., 1963; HARGIS et al., 1968), rats (FREUND et al., 1954), and monkeys (ANDRADA et al., 1969) show a similar response. The fact that the guinea pig responds more readily than other species (LEWIS et al., 1965) is probably due to its pronounced inclination to develop allergic reactions such as anaphylactic shock, tuberculin or delayed hypersensitivity and production of complement fixing components (Figs. 1 and 2).

a) Adjuvants

The introduction of adjuvants in the sensitization procedure has significantly contributed to the potentiation of the natural tissue antigenicity in individuals and in the animal species as a whole. The precise mechanism of the action of adjuvants has not yet been completely clarified, but it is generally accepted that the stimulation of lymphocytic activity and the slow release of the antigen are both necessary for the development of delayed hypersensitivity (RICCI et al., 1969); in addition, the composition and route of injection of the adjuvant are important (FREUND et al., 1953). In this respect, its significant role in the immune response appears to be associated with the formation of a local dermal granuloma which displays macrophages, mononuclear and giant foreign body cells at the site of injection. The *Mycobacterium tuberculosis* or *butyricum*, which constitute together with paraffin oil the complete adjuvant, have a cross reaction with other acid-fast germs. The use of plant oils and other bacteria, such as the nonacid-fast *Corynebacterium rubrum*, may prevent some of the undesirable effects attributed to acid-fast germs (KATSH et al., 1966). These authors also underline the significance of the bound lipids of this microorganism in the induction of the testicular damage. Several reports describing findings related to short- and long-term toxicity of different adjuvants have been published (PECK et al., 1968). It is well known that amyloidosis in the kidney and other organs may be induced by the administration of Freund-type adjuvants (ROTHBARD and WATSON, 1954). It has also been shown that injections of incomplete type of adjuvant (lacking bacteria) together with antigens fail to evoke both testicular and complete immune response (FREUND et al., 1953). Nevertheless, a granuloma similar to that previously referred to may be formed at the dermal site of inoculation. The participation of regional lymph node cells in the sensitization process appears to be of great importance. This is reinforced by the fact that antigens and adjuvants need not necessarily be administered simultaneously; if they are injected separately but on the same side of the animal's back (lymphatic drainage) identical results are obtained (BISHOP, 1961). It would then appear unnecessary that the antigen should be modified at the site of injection (KATSH, 1960 a). Combination of sperm antigen with components of the skin or adjuvant might occur, but such modification is not mandatory since the sperm is regarded as foreign. The more the antigenic configuration of the antigen resembles that of the recipient, the more marked is the tendency to induce the immunologic testicular response (BISHOP, 1961).

b) Antigens of Mature and Immature Testis

According to earlier studies the azoospermic response involved in allergic or immune orchitis is limited to adult animals. However, the antigenic stimulus can be assimilated by very young animals; sensitization soon after birth induces no changes up to the stage of puberty but as soon as testis maturation is completed, aspermatogenesis ensues (BISHOP et al., 1961). Although it has been suggested that gonads of prepuberal animals do not contain the aspermatogenic component, more recent evidence indicates that extracts of immature testes can provoke germinal cell damage, provided that enough material is inoculated (KATSH, 1960 a; POKORNÁ and VÓJTISKOVÁ, 1964 a). To determine the age when the sperm-specific antigens appear, the antigenicity of prepuberal, puberal, and adult rat testis was examined by the double agar gel diffusion technique. It was observed that the testis of 15 day old rats had cross-reacting antigen only with kidney or liver. At 30 days the testis showed one specific antigen not present in other organs, even though no spermatozoa but only spermatids were present. In adult testes, another specific antigen appears, which is identical with testis tissue and sperm cells (ISOJIMA and TIEN SUN LI, 1968). The cell-stage specificity of the testicular response indicates that mature germ cells are autoantigenic, whereas immature germinal tissue is not. Thus, it has been widely admitted according to the recognition concept, that the sperm substance, absent during the tolerant period, fails to register as self and must subsequently be regarded as nonself or foreign and therefore antigenic.

c) Nature of Antigens

Although in the major part of these investigations testicular homogenate was used to sensitize the animals, a more specific and controllable response can be obtained if chemically defined components are used. The complexity of potentially antigenic substances in any one organ and particularly in the testis is not surprising. Antigenicity is physicochemically accepted as an attribute of large molecules with no clear physiologic significance; they can appear as a large variety of molecular entities which may nevertheless evoke a similar tissue response. Testicular homogenate, for instance, as checked by immunoserologic reactions (complement fixation, double agar diffusion, and immunoelectrophoretic tests) reveals a high degree of contamination with other antigens, such as kidney, liver, and serum proteins (SADRI et al., 1967; MARUTA and MOYER, 1967; ALONSO et al., 1969). This heterogeneity of testicular tissue must be taken into consideration when the properties of the corresponding antiserum or the immunologic response are evaluated (Fig. 3). The complexity of the situation is further magnified by the presence of a series of genetically determined factors called histocompatibility antigens, which play an important role in homologous or isologous immunization, though not in the autologous immunization or in inbred animals.

Germinal Cell Antigens. Recently many attempts have been made to isolate and purify the aspermatogenic antigens. Gonads of adult guinea pigs were autoclaved and then submitted to papain and trypsin digestion. Subsequently, different fractions were extracted with trichloroacetic acid, ethanol, and phenol. Inoculation of animals enabled the investigators to conclude that the responsible fraction was thermostable and presumably of a mucopolysaccharide nature (BROWN et al., 1963; BROWN et al., 1965). The application to the testis of various techniques used for the isolation of glycoprotein substances led to the characterization of four glycoprotein substances, which differed with respect to the content of hexosamines, sialic acid, proteins, and lipids. Immunoserologic studies and sensitization of guinea pigs with these materials showed that only two of them reacted with corresponding antisera and also against testis and spermatozoa antisera; no contamination with serum proteins or other tissue proteins was detected (ALONSO et al., 1969).

However, antigenically more potent entities had been extracted earlier from guinea pig testis after ammonium sulphate precipitation, followed by trichloroacetic acid and chloroform. The final product seemed to be a protein-polysaccharide molecule, antigenically active at very low doses (FREUND *et al.,* 1955). Later the study of this complex (a relatively low molecular weight entity, ca. 13,000) was extended, its structure described in detail, and its antigenic power determined at a minimal single dose of 5 μg (BISHOP and CARLSON, 1965; KIRKPATRIC and KATSH, 1964). Enzymatic and electrophoretic methods were employed to study its polypeptide-polysaccharide nature (KATSH and KATSH, 1961) and the inactivation of this antigen by enzymes, tissues, and sera was also attempted. The results obtained can be interpreted to mean that for antigenic activity the following requirements must be met: (a) an 1-amino acid in terminal position and leucine in terminal or near terminal position; (b) the presence of basic amino acids in the polypeptide chain; (c) a beta-glucosidic linkage; (d) 3 – 1,4 linked d-glucose units; (e) a phosphate linked to the lipid; (f) the peptide-sugar-lipid structure must be maintained (KATSH and KATSH, 1966).

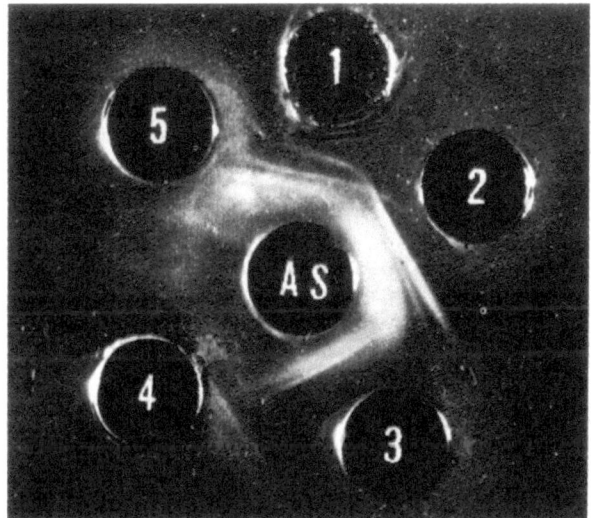

Fig. 3. The heterogenicity of testis tissue and its common antigenicity with other organs and serum proteins as they appear reflected in double agar immunodiffusion technique. (*AS*): anti-guinea pig serum proteins. (*1*): testicular homogenate. (*2*): liver homogenate. (*3*): kidney homogenate (*4*): germinal cells (*5*): thyroid homogenate. Common serum protein antigens are evident in testicular, kidney and liver homogenates. [ALONSO, BUENO, SCACCIATI, GONZALEZ, and MANCINI; Acta europ. Fertil. 1, 459 (1969)]

Important progress in enhancing the antigenic activity was made by the conjugation of this polypeptide-polysaccharide preparation with a hapten, diazosulfonic acid, which induces aspermatogenesis when injected without adjuvant (POKORNÁ and VÓJ-TISKOVÁ, 1964 b). Another testicular component, also aspermatogenic, is the enzyme sorbitol dehydrogenase (BISHOP, 1969), extracted from guinea pig testes and highly purified before administration. This molecule of approximately 105,000 molecular weight appears localized in the mitochondria and cell sap of spermatocytes. Another

enzyme, namely hyaluronidase, has been included among the agents capable of pro-
moting experimental azoospermia (KATSH, 1960 b). Lactic dehydrogenase-X isoenzyme
has also been described as specific for spermatozoa and for meiotic and postmeiotic
spermatogenic cells. Antibodies against auto- and isologous testis in guinea pigs have
been found to exert a selective inhibitory effect upon LDH-X, without influencing
the rest of LDH isoenzymes, which suggests that LDH-X isoenzyme may possess autoantigenic properties (EVREV et al., 1973).

It has been recently demonstrated that a purified preparation of this enzyme is able
to induce aspermatogenesis in homologous immunization in guinea pigs (WELLERSON
et al., 1974).

There is general recognition of the need for further study concerning the identification and characterization of other aspermatogenic antigens, but relatively little has
been published in this area during the last ten years. Formerly, an estimation of the
damage induced in the germinal cells of testis was based on histological grounds, weight
loss of the gland, or decreased number of sperm in the ejaculate; now the use of a
germ-cell specific enzyme, namely sorbitol dehydrogenase, has made possible a
quantitative approach to germinal cell damage provoked by allergic orchitis (BISHOP,
1970).

Table 1. Amino acid analysis of 2 fractions of aspermatogenic antigen. [KATSH, AGUIRRE,
LEAVER and KATSH; Fertil. Steril. 9, 644 (1972)]

	F.2aASA		A.E.ASA	
	μM/mg.	Residues	μM/mg.	Residues
Ala	1.298	12.27	0.587	7.38
Arg	0.414	3.91	0.328	4.10
Asp	0.810	7.65	0.650	8.11
Cys	0.247	2.33	0.397	4.96
Glu	1.482	14.00	0.940	11.85
Gly	0.931	8.78	0.690	8.70
His	0.221	2.09	0.250	3.09
Ile	0.210	1.98	0.190	2.35
Leu	0.489	4.62	0.561	7.01
Lys	1.116	10.55	0.518	6.51
Met	0.144	1.36	0.095	1.19
Phe	0.160	1.51	0.173	2.12
Pro	0.841	7.95	0.733	9.23
Ser	0.848	8.01	0.569	7.22
Thr	0.624	5.90	0.431	5.39
Tyr	0.094	8.88	0.285	3.59
Val	0.653	6.17	0.569	7.18
	Total	107.96	Total	99.98

Table 2. Carbohydrate analysis of 2 fractions of aspermatogenic antigen. (*) Based on anthrone results and carbohydrate distribution by V.P.C. (+) Based on carbohydrate content of 12.67% and molecular weight of 12,600. (‡) Numbers in parenthesis are the nearest integral number of residue. [KATSH et al.; Fertil. Steril. 9, 644 (1972)]

	F.2aASA	A.E.ASA	Molar ratio+
Total neutral sugars (Anthrone)	4.2%	10.46%	
Total sugars	5.07% *	12.67% (V.P.C.)	
Fucose	0.43%	0	

Distribution of monosaccharide residues (as percentage of total carbohydrate)

	F.2aASA	A.E.ASA	Molar ratio+
Fucose	9.26	0	
Mannose	35.31	32.75	2.90 (3)‡
Galactose	30.95	42.15	3.73 (4)
Glucosamine	7.35	0	
N-Acetylglucosamine	12.94	24.94	1.80 (2)
N-Acetylgalactosamine	3.39	0	
N-Acetylneuraminic acid	0.79	0	

More recently (KATSH et al., 1972) another antigen entity has been isolated from the guinea pig testis and reported to be of greater purity than any other yet obtained. Extraction was performed with acetic acid, trichloroacetic acid, and butanol chloroform. Purification was performed by digestion with pepsin and fractionation on Sephadex G-50, followed by precipitation with the corresponding antibody and elution of the antigen-antibody complex. The material thus obtained is antigenically active in microgram amounts when injected with FREUND's complete adjuvant. The purified antigen shows a single band in acrylamide gel and immunoelectrophoresis; it has a molecular weight of 12,600. It is a glycopeptide containing 13% carbohydrate (galactose, mannose, and N-acetylglucosamine). It is probable that the polysaccharide moiety is attached to a polypeptide of 100 residues through N-glycosidic linkage (Tables 1 and 2).

These examples of at least three chemically identified antigenic entities in the guinea pig testis strongly suggest that there is not one aspermatogenic agent, but rather a number of them, which still await clarification as regards their chemical composition, antigenic power, and immunobiological properties. This point will receive more attention below where the antigenicity of sperm cells will be considered.

Nongerminal Cell Antigens. Few investigations have as yet been carried out to ascertain the existence of any immunologic impact upon the testis with antigens originating in nongerminal cell elements. As mentioned before, the immunologic insult in allergic orchitis is germinal cell-stage specific and apparently impairs neither Sertoli and Leydig cells nor seminiferous tubular wall structures. Concurrent with the well-preserved mor-

phology of the Leydig cells, the androgen output of these testes even with severe deple-
tion of germinal epithelium has been found normal. Moreover, the morphology and secretions of the accessory glands appear normal. Nevertheless, more precise data seem to
be needed on androgen synthesis and secretion in allergic orchitis. The selective damage
of the germinative epithelium is also supported by the finding of a higher content of
FSH in the pituitary gland of aspermatogenic guinea pigs; this agrees with the existence of a feedback mechanism between pituitary gonadotropins and the functional germinal epithelium (KATSH and DUNCAN, 1968). Studies on the interstitial tissue reactivity
to immunologic agents are as yet an unexplored field. Concerning this point, attention
must be drawn to the fact that the relative nonantigenicity of steroidal substances has
been overcome by the immune reactions obtained with steroid-protein conjugates; this
suggests the possibility of applying similar methodology in order to inhibit the function of the Leydig cells (BEISER et al., 1959). However, it is evident from recent results
that after active immunization of rabbits with testosterone-protein conjugate, testicular
weight exceeded normal values, and Leydig cells showed an increase in cell volume,
but no damage was apparent in spermatogenesis (NIESCHLAG et al., 1973).

Investigation of the extracellular components (basement membranes and collagen)
of the seminiferous tubular wall is also of considerable biological and immunologic
interest, since these structures are part of the so-called blood-testis barrier (FAWCETT et

Table 3. Amino acid composition and carbohydrate analysis of seminiferous tubule wall component, mainly basement membrane. [DENDUCHIS, LUSTIG, GONZALEZ and MANCINI; Biol. Reprod.
13, 274, 1975]

Amino acid	Residues/ 1000 Residues	Carbohydrates	mg%
Hydroxylysine	20.5	Neutral sugars	3.77
Lysine	44.0	Glucose	1.14
Histidine	16.5	Fucose	0.29
Arginine	48.3	Hexosamines	0.24
Hydroxyproline	63.0	Sialic acid	0.26
Aspartic acid	58.3	Paper chromatography	glu.-gal.-
Threonine	24.9	of neutral sugars	man.-fuc.
Serine	41.4		
Glutamic acid	81.0		
Proline	86.3		
Glycine	199.3		
Alanine	73.4		
Half-cystine	27.3		
Valine	48.1		
Methionine	12.8		
Isoleucine	24.9		
Leucine	51.0		
Tyrosine	15.4		
Phenylalanine	21.3		

al., 1970). Therefore, a preparation of adult rat testis rich in basement membranes showing only few collagen fibers as contaminant, has been isolated and chemically characterized (LUSTIG *et al.*, 1973). The isolation method consisted of several centrifugations
with salt solutions of different molarities, cell disruption by ultrasonic vibration and
enzyme treatment. The high nitrogen content, the presence of sugars and the absence
of lipids suggest that the final material was mostly a glycoprotein. Amino acid and
carbohydrate composition was similar to that obtained for isolated basement membranes from different organs (Table 3). This tubular wall preparation was used as an antigen; rabbits were inoculated and an immune serum of high titer was obtained. Using

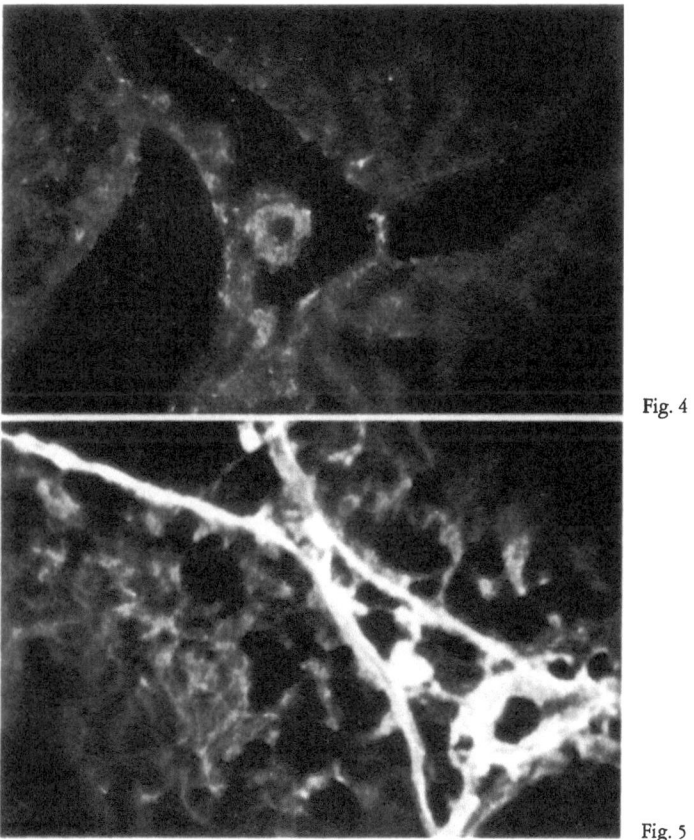

Fig. 4

Fig. 5

Fig. 4. Negative immunofluorescent reaction of seminiferous tubule wall structures. Section of
adult rat testes incubated with normal rabbit globulin followed by goat gamma globulin serum
against rabbit gamma globulins × 180. [LUSTIG, DENDUCHIS, GONZALEZ and MANCINI; Acta Physiol. Latinoamericana 23, 101 (1973)]

Fig. 5. Positive immunofluorescent reaction of seminiferous tubular wall structures. Section of
adult rat testes incubated with rabbit gamma globulin anti-tubule wall components, followed by
labeled goat serum against rabbit gamma globulin. Not only tubule wall appears fluorescent but
also walls of small vessels. Negative reactions in germinal epithelium and Leydig cells. × 180.
[LUSTIG *et al.*; Acta Physiol. Latinoamericana 23, 101 (1973)]

the passive hemagglutination technique, specificity of the immune serum was demonstrated since other related antigens, such as collagen and glycoproteins from germinal cells and from other organs, failed to react (DENDUCHIS et al., 1975).

In vitro and *in vivo* experiments using indirect immunofluorescent and immunoperoxidase techniques, at the light microscope level, showed the antibody localized on the seminiferous tubular wall and not in the other structures of the testis, except for a faint cross-reaction with collagen of the vessel wall. A lack of organ specificity was also demonstrated (Figs. 4 – 5). Preliminary experiments showed that passive immunization of rats with repeated doses of the antiserum injected in the subalbugineal space resulted in the formation of an antigen-antibody complex at seminiferous tubular walls, which subsequently initiated a) inflammatory reaction with polymorphonuclear, macrophage and mononuclear cells, b) weakness of positive PAS reaction normally present in the internal part of tubular walls and c) sloughing of germinal cells (LUSTIG et al., 1976).

Summarizing, it can be postulated that nongerminal cell antigens, other than tubular wall glycoproteins and androgens, might also behave as immunogens capable of causing destruction of germinal elements. Whether this damage results from a primary impact upon these cells, or represents a secondary phenomenon, must be clarified in further experiments.

2. Antigenicity of Spermatozoa

Many efforts have been made in the past to obtain a "toxic" antiserum against sperm cells washed free of seminal plasma. Heterologous, homologous, and even autologous sensitization using rabbits, bulls, guinea pigs, and mice, have all been claimed to be successful (METCHNIKOFF, 1900; GUYER, 1922; KENNEDY, 1924). The antigenicity of spermatozoa was confirmed later on by electrophoretic and serologic methods, with characterization of the immobilizing properties of the corresponding antibodies. These results were achieved by inoculation of rabbits with suspensions of sperm cells from ram, bull, rat, and mouse. Some cross reactions have been obtained with both bull and rabbit sperm antibodies, suggesting the existence of a nondecisive species-specific sperm antigenicity (MUDD and MUDD, 1929; HENLE, 1938). Using ultrasonic vibration and ultracentrifugation, evidence of the existence of three different antigenic activities was presented; the first two thermolabile and located at the level of the head and tail, and a third thermostable, common to both. The antisera exhibited an agglutinating type of reaction specific for each portion of the sperm cell (HENLE et al., 1938).

It was not until the classical work of FREUND et al. (1953), that the auto- and homoantigenicity of guinea pig sperm mixed with complete Freund's adjuvant was clearly demonstrated. In this case, sperm cells obtained from the epididymis were emulsified with the adjuvant, inoculated in a single dose into the back of the animal, and several weeks later the previously described selective damage of the germinal cells duly developed. It was not stated whether the same response could be induced with repeated injections of antigenic material without adjuvant. However, such an assumption seems to be valid since inbred male rats, subcutaneously injected with large quantities of unwashed epididymal spermatozoa without adjuvant, produced humoral antibodies of the agglutinin type. It is also interesting that the presence of this single antibody in the serum does not interfere with either spermatogenesis or fertility of the animal (RÜMKE and TITUS, 1970). In rabbits, homologous sperm cells were able to induce precipitating, agglutinating, and immobilizing antibodies, but no lesions were described in the genital tract (MATSUURA, 1956). Rabbits were also sensitized with homologous epididymal spermatozoa mixed with incomplete Freund's adjuvant. A weak humoral antibody response was observed but no evidence of definite testicular cellular damage. However, positive precipitating antibodies were obtained on inoculating rabbits with guinea pig epididymal sperm (LACOMBE and TEIXEIRA, 1963). Homologous epididymal spermatozoa have also been injected together with Freund's adjuvant, leading to aspermatogenesis in guinea pigs (KATSH, 1959; ISOJIMA and STEPUS, 1959). Following the use of fractionating methods, four antigenic fractions isolated from epididymal spermatozoa, namely hyaluronidase, nucleic acids, polysaccharides, and a protein showing electrophoretic mobility of a globulin, were postulated as being responsible for the aspermatogenic process (KATSH and KATSH, 1961; 1965).

a) Nature of Antigens

Several attempts have been made to isolate and characterize the antigenic properties of different structures of guinea pig epididymal spermatozoa. By means of chemical (CLERMONT et al., 1955) or physical methods (HATHAWAY and HARTREE, 1963) acrosomes were separated from sperm cells; the remaining portion showed under microscopic examination the presence of nucleus, neck and tail. By alcohol precipitation, two fractions were obtained from the acrosome and the remaining portion of sperm, one soluble and the other insoluble. Chemical analysis showed in both the presence of proteins,

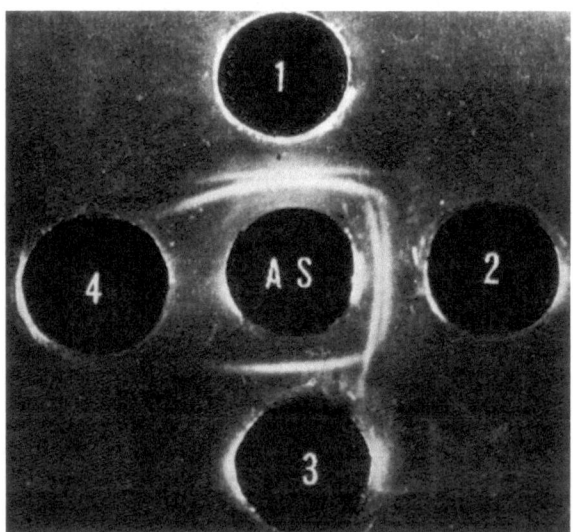

Fig. 6. Double agar diffusion test showing common reactivity between antitesticular serum (*AS*), testis ammonium sulphate fraction (*1*), spermatozoa (*2*) and acrosome (*3*). No lines detectable between antiserum and remaining material from spermatozoa (*4*). [ALONSO et al.; Acta europ. Fertil. 1, 459 (1969)]

lipids, fucose, hexosamines, and sialic acid. The soluble and insoluble fractions of the acrosome showed the highest values in hexosamines and sialic acid, and the remaining portion, which included the nuclei, had a high concentration of lipids, proteins, and nucleic acids. When an immunodiffusion test was applied, it was found that an antitesticular serum reacts positively with spermatozoa and acrosome but not with the remaining portion of sperm; at the same time, common identity was noted for acrosome, spermatozoa, and testicular antigens (Fig. 6). Homologous sensitization of guinea pigs with added Freund's complete adjuvant demonstrated different immunogenic potency of these compounds in terms of antibody response and testicular lesion, the insoluble fraction of acrosome being the highest (MANCINI *et al.*, 1975).

A considerable advance has recently been achieved by the recognition of four different antigens in homogenates of washed epididymal spermatozoa. They have been termed S, P, T and Z. The S, P and T have been isolated and studied (VOISIN and TOULLET, 1968), and the results were as follows: (1) Antigen T is water-soluble, sedimentable at 50,000 g, linked to fragments of cell membranes and possibly lipoproteic in nature. It is thermolabile, destroyed by freeze-drying, periodic acid, trichloroacetic acid, and sodium hydroxide. It is immunogenic and gives rise to autoantibodies, delayed hypersensitivity reactions and testis lesions resembling classical allergic orchitis. (2) Antigen S is soluble in water and trichloroacetic acid and is thermostable. It is a glycoprotein, rich in sugar, with a beta-2 electrophoretic mobility and sucrose gradient centrifugation properties close to those of ovalbumin. It induces both humoral and cellular immunity antibodies and leads to seminiferous tubule lesion. (3) Antigen P is soluble in water, insoluble in trichloroacetic acid and thermostable. It is less sensitive than S to periodate as well as to proteases. It is a protein very poor in sugar, with a beta electrophoretic mobility. As with preceding antigens, it also induces lesions similar to allergic orchitis and both types of antisperm antibodies.

b) Histocompatibility Antigens

There is general agreement that the fate of allogeneic homografts depends on the action of a series of genetically determined factors called histocompatibility antigens (H). For instance, the estimated number of these antigens for skin and spleen grafts is around fifteen. There are differences in activity among the histocompatibility antigens, and they are carried predominantly by spleen, lymph node cells, and leukocytes (BARNES, 1964). As regards the sperm cells, the numerous positive results of tests for H-antigens made with mouse and human spermatozoa, are fairly convincing. The demonstration of such antigens on spermatozoa depends on serologic tests, hemagglutination, cytotoxic antibody assay, immunofluorescent methodology, and inhibition of skin homografts. A fundamental problem concerns the existence of these H-antigens in precursor diploid cells. Their origin through adsorption on the cell surface might be invoked as a possibility, for other antigens of the ABO system and the so-called "coating antigens" are believed to be incorporated in this way into human sperm. Recent findings using inhibition of hemagglutination and indirect immunofluorescence indicate that H-2 antigens are present on testicular cells which do not include haploid spermatogenic elements. Immunofluorescent localization displays a distribution of antigens confined to primary spermatocytes, while spermatogonia as well as nonspermatogenic cells appear negative (VÓJTISKOVÁ and POKORNÁ, 1971). These results have been extended by immunofluorescent and radioactive antiglobulin tests on spermatozoa, which showed a distribution of H-2 antigens on the head and mid-piece of mouse spermatozoa. Experiments in which lymphocytes and spermatozoa were mixed suggest that

the latter possess about 1/10 the amount of H-antigens of the former. Confirming earlier claims, no evidence for haploid expression of these antigens on spermatozoa has
been found (ERICKSON, 1971).

3. Antigenicity of Seminal Plasma

Early work has shown that washed spermatozoa or whole semen may induce in heterologous immunization high titers of sperm immobilizing antibodies. More recent investigations (RAO and SADRI, 1960) emphasize the complexity of semen and the need to consider sperm and seminal plasma antigens separately. The high antigenic potency of seminal plasma obtained by centrifugation of whole semen has been repeatedly confirmed. Serologic techniques and immunoelectrophoresis have disclosed the existence of several fractions which immunologically are common to serum proteins, epididymal and prostate fluids.

a) Antigenic Components

In guinea pig seminal plasma eleven antigenic fractions have been identified, two or three of which belong to serum proteins and the remaining ones are related to spermatozoal antigens (PERNOT and SZUMOWSKI, 1958). Guinea pig seminal plasma has three different components as shown by the ultracentrifugal pattern, but no further studies have been made with regard to antigenicity (SHULMAN and ORSINI, 1970).

Bull seminal plasma injected into rabbits and examined by double agar diffusion technique shows sixteen different antigens, six of which belong to serum proteins and four to sperm cells (RAO and SADRI, 1960). Ejaculated rabbit semen shows nine antigens, seven of which are related to seminal plasma, two to blood serum and two appear to be sperm-specific, originating in the testis (MENGE and PROTZMAN, 1967). Ultracentrifugal studies of rabbit seminal plasma show a prominent 1.85 S peak with a 4.20 S shoulder and minor fast components. Subjected to molecular sieving through Sephadex G-100, it shows marked heterogeneity; five fractions have been defined which contain several macromolecular components as demonstrated by polyacrylamide gel electrophoresis, agar gel immunoelectrophoresis and immunodiffusion assays (YANTORNO et al., 1972).

Immunodiffusion and immunoelectrophoresis of ram seminal plasma indicate distinctly the presence of globulins in beta-2 and beta-globulin positions. The immunoglobulin content was found to be about 2% of that in blood serum (JOHNSON and SETCHELL, 1968). As regards the antigenic components, ram seminal plasma shows nine water-soluble precipitable antigens, which may be reduced to four, if absorption with blood serum is performed (BRATANOV et al., 1973). In contrast to some reports, the finding of specific seminal plasma antigens has been corroborated by direct and cross-immunoserologic reaction (HUNTER, 1969; MARUTA and MOYER, 1967). Contrary to the claim that all ram sperm antigens are related to those of ram seminal plasma (HATHAWAY and HARTREE, 1963), this semen contains at least three antigens inducing auto- and isoantibody formation, one of them being present in spermatozoa, the other in the seminal plasma and the third in both materials (BRATANOV et al., 1973). It is thus highly probable that during transit sperm cells are firmly coated with strongly antigenic material from seminal plasma constituents (WEIL, 1965). This assumption is reinforced by the fact that repeated washing of spermatozoa considerably lessens their antigenic potency (MOYER and MARUTA, 1967).

b) Antigenic Potency

Antigenicity of seminal plasma has also been demonstrated in boars and rabbits by the induction of isoimmune and autoimmune serum, tested by double diffusion and hemagglutination techniques. It is interesting to note that in these experiments the sperm immobilizing test yielded negative results with the immune serum to homologous spermatozoa, and that spermatogenesis was not affected in male animals carrying these antibodies in serum (VESELSKY and MATOUSEK, 1973). On the other hand, it has been reported that rabbit seminal plasma is weakly antigenic in the homologous sensitization procedure (STEVENS and FOST, 1964). Immunologic studies on organ specificity using heteroantisera showed that rabbit seminal plasma contains a mixture of genital-tract-specific antigens and several antigens shared with other organs and serum. Using selected autoantisera, the presence was demonstrated of two distinct auto-antigens specific to the rabbit accessory glands and additional autoantigens from testis and/or epididymis, proving the complex autoantigenic nature of rabbit seminal plasma (YANTORNO et al., 1972). The possibility that seminal plasma induces lesions of an allergic orchitis type in the rabbit and guinea pig has been questioned (WEIL and FINKLER, 1958; VULCHANOV, 1969). However, chemically modified rabbit seminal plasma preparations, in which the proteins were coupled to diazonium derivatives of sulphanilic acid, or even native seminal plasma, together with Freund's adjuvant, were used to inoculate homologous animals. Serologic tests such as hemagglutination, sperm immobilization, skin test and Ouchterlony technique were positive at varying intervals of time. A depression in the sperm count and lesions similar to those of allergic orchitis were found in the testis (YANTORNO et al., 1971). Further studies are needed to identify the protein fraction responsible for the antigenicity of the whole seminal plasma.

4. Antigenicity of Male Accessory Glands

A number of tissues have been studied in the past with respect to their organ-specific antigens. In many instances it has been possible to produce autoantibodies against characteristic components. The testis, epididymis, and seminal plasma have been largely explored from this angle.

Interest in the field of accessory glands began many years ago, when the first cross-reactions between extracts of prostate, seminal vesicles and seminal plasma were demonstrated. As a consequence, the possibility that some seminal plasma antigens might be present in the accessory glands before being secreted into the genital tract opened up a new approach to possible autoimmunologic damage of these glands and of seminal spermatozoa as well. Saline extracts of prostatic secretion from bulls, tested by double agar diffusion technique preceded by absorption of nonspecific precipitins, showed four antigens common to serum proteins and spermatozoa. The seminal vesicles have been found to have three to five antigens, also with common reactivity to spermatozoa (RAO and SADRI, 1959). Homologous antiserum against seminal vesicle secretion could also be obtained in rabbits, and gel precipitation procedure gave only one line when tested against its own antiserum, and none against testis antiserum (AB-REU et al., 1963). Attempts were made to induce cross-immunologic damage in the testis by repeated immunization of mice with epididymal extracts (free of sperm) plus adjuvant; it was claimed that spermatogenesis was adversely affected and fertility of females markedly reduced after mating with immunized males (SETHYE and RAO, 1968). Isoimmunization with extracts of rabbit male accessory glands, administered with complete Freund's adjuvant, has been found to induce a specific autoantibody response as well as delayed hypersensitivity. In these animals, tissue damage was observed in all the accessory glands while the kidneys and testes remained virtually normal. Lesions were mainly represented by mononuclear infiltration and flattening or desquamation of the epithelial cells. Comparable results were obtained as before mentioned, with either native or chemically modified seminal plasma, although in this case testicular damage was also usually recorded (YANTORNO et al., 1973).

a) Prostate Gland

Systematic studies on the antigenicity and immunologic behavior of accessory glands have demonstrated that autoantibodies to the male accessory tissues of reproduction could be produced in rabbits by intensive immunization using saline extracts of rabbit prostate gland or, as noted above, of the total complex of accessory glands. Although the prostate was considered of major significance, it has been shown that the autoantigenic material in this tissue is shared by the seminal vesicles, coagulating gland and bulbo-urethral gland (SHULMAN *et al.*, 1966). Such material was also found in the seminal plasma, but evidence showed that this was due to admixture of fluids from the accessory tissues, and was absent from other sites of the urogenital tract, such as kidney, bladder, testis, and epididymis. As it is also absent from prostatic tissue of other species, the antigen was considered to possess a high degree of species-specificity.

Immunodiffussion studies of this tissue suggested that two antigens were present, as judged by the appearance of two lines which were close together. It also seems that another two antigens may be elicited in homologous sensitization in rabbits, if ethanol-resistant preparations are used. The accessory glands of the sensitized animals did not show histological damage, in spite of high hemagglutinating antibody titers (SHULMAN *et al.*, 1966). Further studies of this group have demonstrated that dog prostatic fluid injected into rabbits induced antibodies containing at least three components as revealed by immunodiffussion, with different molecular weight and antigenic properties (SHULMAN and AHMED, 1971). Guinea pigs immunized with homogenates prepared with prostate gland plus complete adjuvant developed a cross reaction between this gland and spermatozoa (CHERNYSHOV and PODOPLELOV, 1973). Antibodies which became more reactive after adsorption of spermatozoa with prostatic fluid could be demonstrated; cross-reactions with serum proteins and other organ antigens were also detected.

b) Seminal Vesicles

Homo- and autoantibodies against seminal vesicle fluid have been produced in male and female guinea pigs as shown by hemagglutination and precipitation methods (VULCHANOV, 1969). A more detailed biochemical study demonstrated that guinea pig seminal vesicle fluid is homogeneous by ultracentrifugal analysis, revealing a single boundary with a sedimentation coefficient of 1.55. In contrast, electrophoretic separation methods indicated six components, three of which were major components of approximately equal proportions. One of these components was shown to be strongly antigenic in heteroimmunization tests, whereas the others failed to show any antigenicity. By procedures of isoimmunization in guinea pigs, this component was also found to be immunogenic, giving rise to autoantibodies in the male. The majority of the animals exhibited positive skin tests and many had tissue lesions consisting of interstitial infiltration of mononuclear cells with evident alteration of tubular epithelium (ORSINI and SHULMAN, 1971). In connection with the biological properties of these accessory gland antibodies, it was also reported that agglutination of guinea pig sperm *in vitro* may be induced by an antiserum against prostate or seminal vesicle, but with a lower titer compared to that against epididymis (MARUTA and MOYER, 1967).

In short, evidence seems to indicate that sperm-specific as well as seminal plasma-specific antigens may cross react with others from the accessory glands, but it remains to be seen which of these are implicated in the impairment of fertilizing capacity of spermatozoa.

5. Antibodies

It is generally admitted that in a given immunologic system the antibodies formed may be of many types but are substantially classified into two categories. The first comprises those called humoral or circulating antibodies, predominantly formed by plasmocytes; they may be detected by their ability to develop local or general anaphylaxis, to fix complement, to agglutinate antigen-coated red cells by immunoelectrophoresis, precipitation curves, and *in vitro* lysis of target cells (cytotoxic effect). The second, preferentially named cellular immunity, corresponds to the classical fixed or cell bound antibodies (delayed hypersensitivity); it is mediated by lymphocytes and the result is the final damage of tissue by a mechanism in direct contact with the effector cells. These antibodies are mainly tested by the delayed classical skin test, *in vitro* inhibition of macrophage migration and blastoid transformation of leukocytes. Therefore, in evaluating the reaction against any antigen, all antibodies belonging to these two types must be tested.

a) Humoral Antibodies

We have already described above how testis, sperm cells, seminal plasma or accessory gland antigens added with complete adjuvants are capable of inducing the so-called antisperm antibodies. In this system it is possible to identify an immune response characterized by different types of humoral antibodies and cellular immunity as well, the latter being more constantly present and more closely related to tissue damage than the former. As only a single injection with added adjuvant is required to obtain the typical immune orchitis, some investigators have tried to demonstrate that the characteristics of primary and secondary sensitization to homologous spermatozoa or seminal plasma conform to the antibody response produced with other antigens and in various species; thus, a single injection of the antigen following the decline of serum antibodies after the primary response is responsible for a higher peak and longer duration of antibody titers (MOYER and MARUTA, 1967). It has been stated that the various kinds of antibodies formed would depend on the individual animal, the method used, and the route of sensitization (CHUTNÁ and RYCHLIKOVÁ, 1964 a; BISHOP and CARLSON, 1965).

In the case of guinea pig testis or sperm antigens injected by cutaneous route, a homogenate was more frequently used than chemical fractions or specific chemical entities to induce sperm antibodies and the allergic or immunologic orchitis.

Anaphylaxis. In the guinea pig the humoral antibodies are related to the general sensitization of the animal and are expressed by the typical anaphylactic shock if a minimal dose of the antigen alone is intravenously injected. Local immediate anaphylaxis may also be seen when an intradermal injection of a small amount of antigen alone is given. It consists of a wheal-like response, which develops in 1 – 2 hours and histologically corresponds to dermal congestive vessels and exudation of polymorphonuclear leukocytes (FREUND *et al.*, 1953 – 1955). These types of antibodies may also be passively demonstrated by injecting intradermally the immune serum into the dermis of a homologous receptor (passive cutaneous anaphylaxis, PCA). Several hours after inoculation, a small dose of testicular antigen together with Trypan blue as indicator of vascular permeability is intravenously injected. As a result of the antigen-antibody interaction, the site of dermal injection develops an acute inflammation and a blue spot of variable dimensions.

Complement Fixing. These antibodies also appear (endpoint 50% hemolysis) and can be demonstrated by using as antigen the supernatant of tissue homogenate in a dilution of about 1/400. Titers in general are low, ranging from 1/64 to 1/320.

Precipitins. Precipitating types as shown by the old capillary method or by the modern double agar diffusion technique are a less frequent antibody, detectable after sensitization with testis antigens, and which appear as one or two lines at most.

Hemagglutinins. The passive hemagglutination technique has been seldom used in animals immunized with testis homogenate. Results may appear positive at low or moderate titer using as antigen the supernatant of tissue homogenate.

Immobilisins. Although normal homologous or heterologous serum immobilizes sperm cells *in vitro*, the immune serum of sensitized animals does so at much higher titers, ranging from 1/16 to 1/128. This property is complement dependent, but the specificity of the effect and the precise immunologic characteristic of the responsible factor in guinea pig serum need clarification (CHANG, 1947; MANCINI *et al.*, 1969).

Cytotoxins. Closely related to this immunologic activity is the lytic effect on the acrosome of spermatozoa and spermatids, also present in normal homologous serum (SPOONER, 1964). Swelling of acrosome and the loss of PAS reaction, normally present in this structure, characterize the lytic effect as follows: (1) the appearance of empty areas in the peripheral zone of acrosome; (2) increased number of vesicles and (3) loosening of subcellular particles in the cytoplasm and in the chromatin of the nuclei of developing spermatids (MANCINI *et al.*, 1969) (Figs. 7 – 9). These studies have been extended recently. A selective antibody against one of the antigens, present in the external membrane of the sperm acrosome (antigen T) and easily accessible to antibodies, has been claimed to be responsible for the lytic action (LE BOUTELIER *et al.*, 1973). Striking changes consisting of regularly spaced 60 – 200 Å holes through which acrosomal material exuded have been detected in the outer membrane of rabbit spermatozoa (RUSSO and METZ, 1974). This effect, also complement dependent and probably localized in the IgG_2 fraction, corresponds to the original and classical concept, whereby antibody and complement act on the cell membrane, where they produce a permeability disorder which induces the loss of low molecular weight constituents from the cells and equilibration of cations between cells and the medium (GREEN and SILVERBLATT,

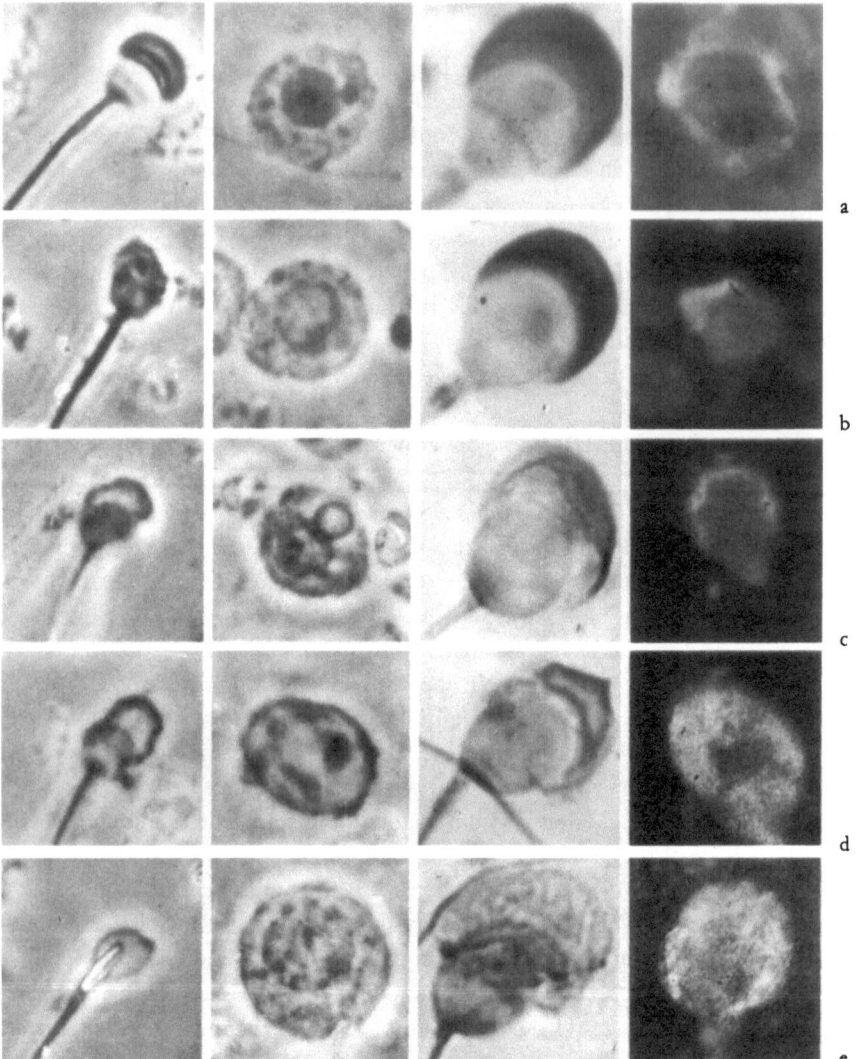

Fig. 7. Grouped in four columns and identified from top to bottom as: a, b, c, d, e. All cells belong to adult guinea pigs. × 900. *First column:* spermatozoa as seen in phase microscopy. a) normal sperm incubated with normal homologous serum plus complement; compact and homogenous acrosome. b), c), d), and e) normal sperm incubated with homologous antitestis serum plus complement; marked swelling and disruption of acrosome. *Second column:* a) spermatid incubated with normal homologous serum plus complement; no signs of alteration visible. b), c), and d) spermatids incubated with antitestis serum plus complement; swelling of cytoplasm and nuclei. e) spermatocyte incubated with antitestis serum plus complement; no alteration is detectable. *Third column:* a) and b) spermatozoa incubated with normal homologous serum plus complement. PAS reaction. Uniform staining of the acrosome. c), d), and e) spermatozoa incubated with antitestis serum plus complement. PAS reaction. Weak or absent reactivity of acrosome which appears vacuolated and distorted. *Fourth column:* a), b), and c) spermatids incubated with homologous antitestis serum followed by labeled rabbit globulin anti guinea pig gamma globulin. Immunofluorescent technique. Staining of the perinuclear acrosome granule or area. d) and e) spermatozoa incubated as above. Intense reactivity of acrosome area; no staining in remaining structures [MANCINI, MONASTIRSKY, FERNÁNDEZ, COLLAZO, SEIGUER, and ALONSO; Fertil. Steril. **20**, 779 (1969)]

1960). This may be demonstrated by the intracellular penetration of a dye or by the sensitive radioactive technique using labeled chromium as indicator of cell permeability. The application of this test to the antisperm system has been performed with eosin as vital dye (JOHNSON, 1970 a).

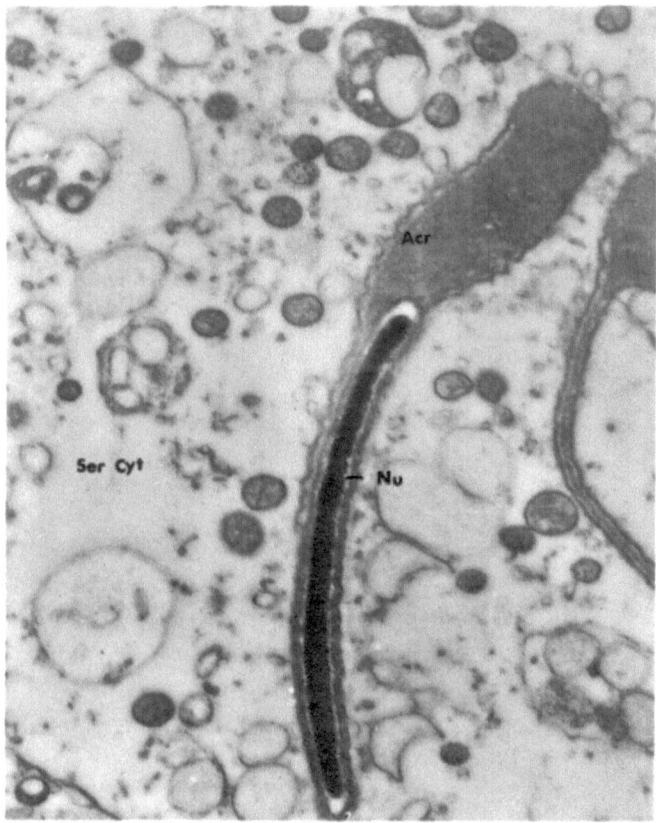

Fig. 8. Testicular spermatozoa incubated with homologous serum plus complement. No gross modifications observable in the acrosome (*Acr*) and nucleus (*Nu*). Fragments of Sertoli cell cytoplasm also seen (*Ser Cyt*) Electron micrograph. × 8,000 [MANCINI *et al.*; Fertil. Steril. 20, 779 (1969)]

Agglutinins. Another type of activity may be present in immune sera, namely the agglutinating effect on previously immobilized spermatozoa as shown by the capillary tube test. There is no complement dependence and it is probably related to an immunoglobulin fraction. At low titer this activity is demonstrable in normal serum, but titers increase markedly in guinea pigs sensitized with homologous testis antigen applied with complete Freund's adjuvant. No correlation has yet been made between this test and other parameters in allergic orchitis (SHULMAN *et al.*, 1971). As stated earlier, this agglutination property is also induced in syngeneic rats by inoculation with large

quantities of spermatozoa without adjuvant, but no correlation with damage of spermatogenesis has been established (RÜMKE and TITUS, 1970).

Cytophilic Activity. Cytophilic activity (BOYDEN and SORKIN, 1961) was recently found in serum of guinea pigs sensitized with testicular homogenate plus adjuvant

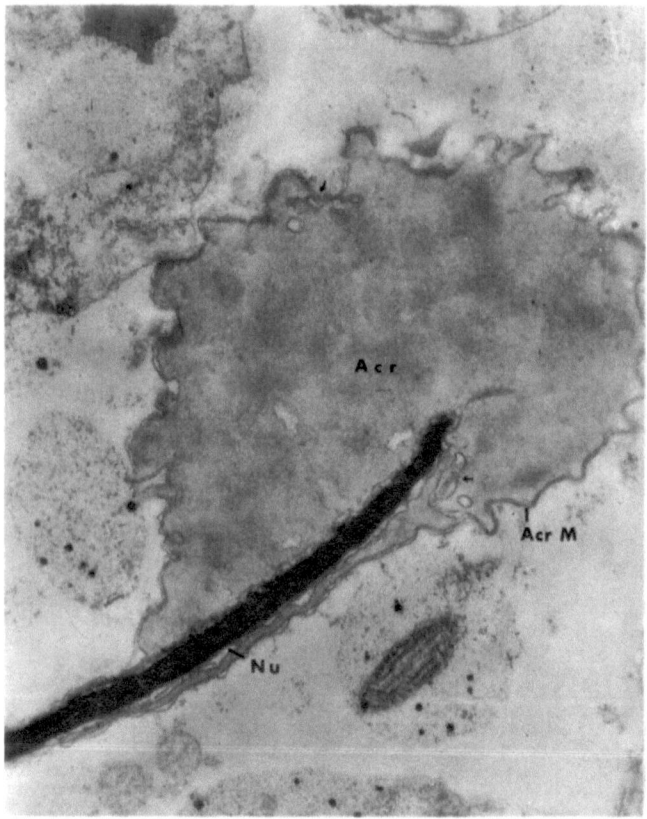

Fig. 9. Testicular sperm incubated with homologous antitestis serum plus complement, Hypertrophy of the acrosoma (*Acr*), numerous infoldings (*arrow at top*) of acrosome membrane (*Acr
M*) and areas of low electron-density adjacent to the inner membrane of acrosome; nucleus is apparently normal. Cellular debris from surrounding germinal elements are also seen. Electron-micrograph. × 18,000. [MANCINI *et al.*; Fertil. Steril. 20, 779 (1969)]

(MAZZOLLI and BARRERA, 1974). This new property of antisperm serum confers upon
macrophages from the peritoneal cavity of normal sensitized guinea pigs the ability to
adsorb *in vitro* homologous or own spermatozoa. There is no complement dependence
of this activity and specificity is substantiated by the fact that other peritoneal cells,
such as leukocytes or red cells, do not attach spermatozoa to their surface. A "natural
cytophilic activity" is also present at low levels in normal serum; in both cases the
IgG_2 globulin fraction seems to be responsible (BARRERA *et al.*, 1976). The significance
of this activity is probably related to phagocytosis, as suggested in other immune sys-

tems (BERKEN and BENACERRAF, 1966). Such cytophilic activity was found in the sera of guinea pigs from eight days onward, after sensitization with testis homogenate in complete Freund's adjuvant. Only low and transitory levels were found in a few animals when antigen was administered together with incomplete adjuvant (Fig. 10).

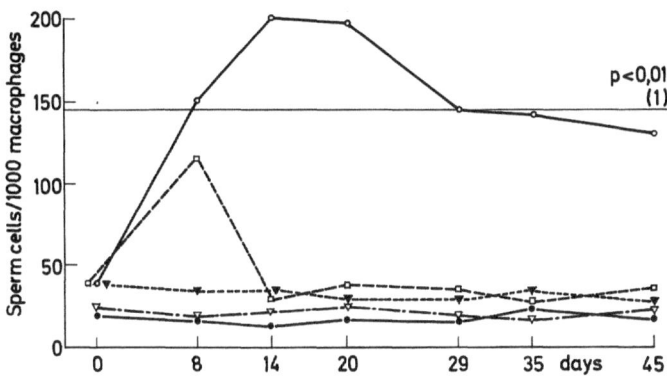

Fig. 10. Variations of cytophylic activity in serum of guinea pigs after immunization with testis antigens plus complete Freund's adjuvant. As control, other animals were sensitized with antigen or complete or incomplete adjuvant alone. [MAZZOLLI and BARRERA; J. Immunol. Methods 4, 41 (1974)]

Testicular homogenate plus complete Freund's adjuvant ─────────
Testicular homogenate plus incomplete Freund's adjuvant ──────────
Kidney homogenate plus complete Freund's adjuvant ··············
Complete Freund's adjuvant ─·─·─·─·─·─·─·
Testicular homogenate alone ─────────

Although there are no precise data on the time sequence of the appearance of the different antibodies described above, it is generally agreed that most of them are detectable during the second week and tend to disappear around the sixth week after sensitization.

Immunofluorescent Antibody. There has been no clear demonstration of an effective increase in the level of endogenous gamma globulin in allergic orchitis. However, some reports claim that a deposition of this globulin may be shown in the peritubular tissue and inside the seminiferous tubule using the immunofluorescent method (BROWN et al., 1953). While some authors using this technique have reported negative findings in seminiferous tubules (MANCINI et al., 1964), others have demonstrated by autoradiography a passage of I–125 labeled immune IgG only into the canaliculi of the rete testis and straight tubules (TUNG et al., 1970). When the double immunofluorescent technique is applied to sections of testis, epididymis, or to smears of spermatozoa, it has been repeatedly shown that an antiacrosomal factor is present in the gamma globulin fraction of the antiserum. The acrosome or precursor organelles present in earlier spermatids and in spermatozoa appear uniformly and brilliantly stained, but no reaction is observable in spermatocytes, spermatogonia, or Sertoli cells (Fig. 7). The reaction is negative in immature testis or damaged gonads lacking spermiogenic cells.

As this result was obtained in guinea pigs, rats and mice sensitized with testicular homogenate, it may be deduced that the acrosome contains the antigen or antigens implicated in the antigenic potency of the testis and the sperm cells (BAUM, 1959; SWANSON et al., 1962; MANCINI et al., 1962; BARTH and RUSSEL, 1964).

It is interesting to stress that the complement factor is usually involved in several of the immunobiological reactions of antitesticular or antispermatozoal and normal sera (EDWARDS, 1960). As normal guinea pig serum possesses at lower titer the ability to immobilize or lyse sperm cells and even reacts with the acrosome by the immunofluorescent technique, an attempt was made to characterize immunochemically this naturally occurring antisperm antibody. It was shown that after ultracentrifugation all antispermatozoal activity was in the 7S fraction which corresponds to the fast gamma globulin, following distribution from column fractionation procedures. It was proved, using antiserum against C_3 component of complement, that fluorescence was also confined to the acrosome, but was no longer detectable if serum was adequately treated in order to remove complement (JOHNSON, 1968). Thus, complement fixation, immunofluorescence, and other tests have demonstrated low titer positive reactions between spermatozoa and serum from normal animals. This factor is absent in young animals, but appears at puberty and can be absorbed out with sperm or testis extract. Whether these immunologic reactions detect the same fraction in serum and the mechanism of the formation of this antisperm factor under normal conditions are problems still to be solved (EDWARDS, 1963).

It is worthwhile to recall that not all the animals sensitized with different testis or sperm antigens reacted with similar antibody response. For instance, the antigenic difference between whole autoclaved testis and the subsequent papainized material is illustrated when sera of these two series of animals are compared. PCA reaction is only obtained with sera of guinea pigs immunized with whole testis. There is also a lack of correlation between the PCA test and the demonstration in the seminiferous tubules of endogenous circulating globulins, which might be due to the production of different proportions of 19S and 7S antibodies. This lack of correlation also extends to the sperm immobilization test and to the damage of germinal cells (BROWN et al., 1963). Moreover, anti-testis or anti-ASPM (ammonium sulphate-precipitated fraction from testis homogenate) guinea pig serum reacts by double agar diffusion or immunoelectrophoresis either with testis homogenate or ASPM, but not with TCA (trichloroacetic acid fraction) or CPM complex (polysaccharide component). On the other hand, all three fractions give positive PCA tests against antitestis or anti-ASPM sera. These results may be due to the recognized higher sensitivity of the PCA method, to the fact that CPM would be altered or stripped of some reactive groups during extraction, or to the presence of both antibodies only in the anti-ASPM serum (BISHOP and CARLSON, 1965). In the same sense extracts of germinal cells, acrosome, or a glycoprotein isolated from guinea pig sperm cells react positively in the complement fixation test against antitesticular serum, but are negative in the agar diffusion technique (ALONSO et al., 1969).

A more detailed study of the various antibodies depending on the antigens used and their localization on globulin fractions and reactions with different parts of guinea pig spermatozoa was recently provided (VOISIN and TOULLET, 1968). Antigen T (description above) induces complement fixing, cytotoxic and cellular immunity antibodies. By immunofluorescence it appears localized in the acrosomic granule and head cap of spermatozoa. Antigen S gives rise to low complement fixing titers (IG_2), autoantibodies capable of inducing PCA and hemagglutinating positive tests and strong delayed hypersensitivity, but not those of a precipitating or spermotoxic type. These antibodies have been found to be essentially IG_1 anaphylactic type; by immunofluorescence they react with proacrosomal and acrosomal granules of spermatids and the acrosome of spermatozoa. Antigen P is more complex than antigen T, for the antibodies formed are both of anaphylactic and complement fixing types. Both antigens are also of a precipitating type, giving rise to passive hemagglutination and inducing immediate and delayed hypersensitivity; they show cytotoxic properties in the presence of complement fixing activity (TOULLET et al., 1973).

Although several authors have denied the possibility of getting allergic orchitis by immunization with seminal plasma (WEIL and FINKLER, 1958; STEVENS and FOST, 1964), recent studies favor the hypothesis that this antigen may not only evoke antisperm antibodies but also lesions of testis in guinea pigs (VULCHANOV, 1969) and in rabbits (YANTORNO et al., 1971). Animals sensitized with whole seminal plasma plus Freund's adjuvant showed positive hemagglutinating titer but only when seminal plasma, and not testis extract, was used as a challenge antigen. On the other hand, the immune serum gives positive reaction with testicular extract by complement fixation and agar diffusion tests. Likewise, sperm immobilizing activity was found in sera from animals of all groups. Delayed skin test appeared positive against testicular extract only in animals inoculated with chemically modified seminal plasma, and also in all animals challenged with extracts of accessory glands (YANTORNO et al., 1971).

b) Cellular Immunity

As regards the cellular immunity (delayed hypersensitivity, fixed or cell bound antibodies), the involvement of lymphocytes (circulating B and T lymphocytes) in the cellular transfer of altered tissue reactivity and their participation in apparently diverse functions, such as immunologic surveillance of neoplastic cells, rejection of homografts and mediation of certain autoimmune diseases, emphasize the immunologic response mediated by this population of cells, thus providing a new tool for examining the mechanism of production of immunologic diseases (LAWRENCE, 1969). It is also generally accepted that macrophages participate in some manner in the interaction with lymphocytes. Phagocytic activity of the antigen may result in the formation of an immunogenic complex bound to macrophage RNA, which ultimately is transferred to lymphocytes as informational RNA for the synthesis of specific antibodies (FISHMAN et al., 1973). Until recently an accepted characteristic of cell-mediated immunity has been the requirement of living lymphoid cells, rather than a product derived from them, in the initiation of the specific type of inflammatory response which ultimately results in tissue damage. However, a long series of more recent experiments has demonstrated that substances of a polypeptide nature, liberated by these cells in the presence of antigens *in vitro,* and also probably of effector cells in the *in vivo* system, are responsible for the damage induced (LAWRENCE and VALENTINE, 1970; GRANGER, 1970).

Application of these concepts to allergic orchitis has proved that at least two tests mediated by these cells appear positive, the classical skin test and the *in vitro* inhibition of migration of macrophages. Injection of a minute amount of testicular antigen alone into animals sensitized with testis antigens plus complete adjuvant provokes in 24 – 48 hrs a dermal reaction expressed by proliferation of histiocytes and fibroblasts, edema, hypertrophy of vascular endothelium, and accumulation of mononuclear round cells around vessels. It is generally agreed that papules 5 – 8 mm in diameter develop on the 6th day after sensitization and persist for several months (FREUND *et al.,* 1953). Chronologically, the humoral antibody appears later, around the 9th – 12th day, while testis lesion starts between the 10th – 12th day. As with humoral antibodies, it will depend on the antigen used whether a correlation between the skin test, humoral antibody and testis lesion will occur in the more advanced stages of the disease (BROWN *et al.,* 1963; BISHOP, 1970). It is interesting to recall that rabbits sensitized with seminal plasma plus complete adjuvant develop a positive skin test when challenged with an extract of accessory glands, while only those injected with chemically modified seminal plasma react to testicular homogenate (YANTORNO *et al.,* 1971).

The inhibition of macrophage migration is based on the ability of the antigen to prevent the migration of macrophages obtained from the peritoneal exudate of sensitized animals (GEORGE and VAUGHAN, 1962). This method has two great advantages, namely the ability to reproduce results regardless of skin reactivity and the possibility of obtaining quantitative data. It has recently been reported that cells in the peritoneal exudate obtained from guinea pigs within seven days after sensitization with testis homogenate plus adjuvant exhibit inhibition of migration when cultured in the presence of supernatant of testicular homogenate. It appears that this test, if adequately controlled, may detect earlier than the skin test the delayed hypersensitivity reaction (MAZZOLLI, 1971). No data as yet exist concerning either the *in vitro* blastoid transformation of lymphocytes from sensitized animals in the presence of testicular antigen, or the immunobiological effect of lymphocyte soluble factors on germinal epithelium.

It is obvious that further investigations are needed to establish a closer correlation between different types of antibodies and different antigens in this immune system. The effect of immunoglobulin fractions and lymphocyte soluble factors with a given immunobiological property, that is cytotoxic, hemagglutinating, complement fixing, precipitating, delayed hypersensitivity, and germinal cell lesions should also be studied. The use of purified antigens instead of entire testicular homogenates will undoubtedly help the understanding of this autoimmune condition.

6. Histopathology

In general the histology of the immunologic orchitis is now considered to represent a true orchiepididymitis, affecting the canaliculi of the different portions of epididymis, ductus efferent, rete testis, and seminiferous tubules (Figs. 11 – 14). The observations made (WAKSMAN, 1959 a; BROWN *et al.,* 1963; MANCINI, 1964; JOHNSON, 1970 a) align the experimental orchitis with other experimental auto-allergies which affect the central and peripheral nervous system, the lens, uvea of the eye, the thyroid and the adrenal.

a) Light Microscopy

Several studies have reported similar histological lesions in the testis of the rat (FREUND *et al.,* 1954), mouse (POKORNÁ *et al.,* 1963; HARGIS *et al.,* 1968), monkey (ANDRADA *et al.,* 1969), and rabbit (YANTORNO *et al.,* 1972), but most of the work refers to guinea pigs immunized with testis homogenate, testis antigens, or sperm cells, administered with complete Freund's adjuvant. So far, there is still controversy concerning the time sequence of events detectable in the seminiferous tubules and intertubular spaces. According to some investigators (WAKSMAN, 1959 a; TUNG *et al.,* 1970) the lesion appears to be secondary to an inflammatory disease and is found to consist of earlier disseminated foci of perivenous inflammation; lymphocytes and histiocytes predominate in the cellular infiltrate with later invasion of epididymal, rete and seminiferous tubule epithelium, and destruction of germinal cells, leaving intact Leydig and Sertoli cells.

Observations made two weeks after sensitization of guinea pigs with autoclaved testis have shown that, while some areas of the testis are affected, others are damaged slightly or not at all. Cellular infiltration, histiocytes, fibroblasts, and mononuclear cells, mainly lymphocytes, are sometimes present, but affected tubules are infrequently associated with infiltration. The epididymis contains sperm and some degenerated germ cells but no intercanalicular infiltration is seen. During the third week there is almost complete loss of cells in some seminiferous tubules and infiltration of inflammatory cells in the interstitium may be present. The proximal portion of epididymis is devoid of sperm, but sperm is still found in the distal segment; some patchy infiltration of leukocytes in the intercanalicular space can also be seen. At four weeks, the seminiferous tubules appear almost empty of germinal cells and infiltration is variable. Sperm cells are still present in the distal epididymis and accumulation of mononuclear cells is apparent. By the sixth week there are no germinal cells visible, Leydig cells appear morphologically normal and intertubular infiltration is absent. Regeneration of

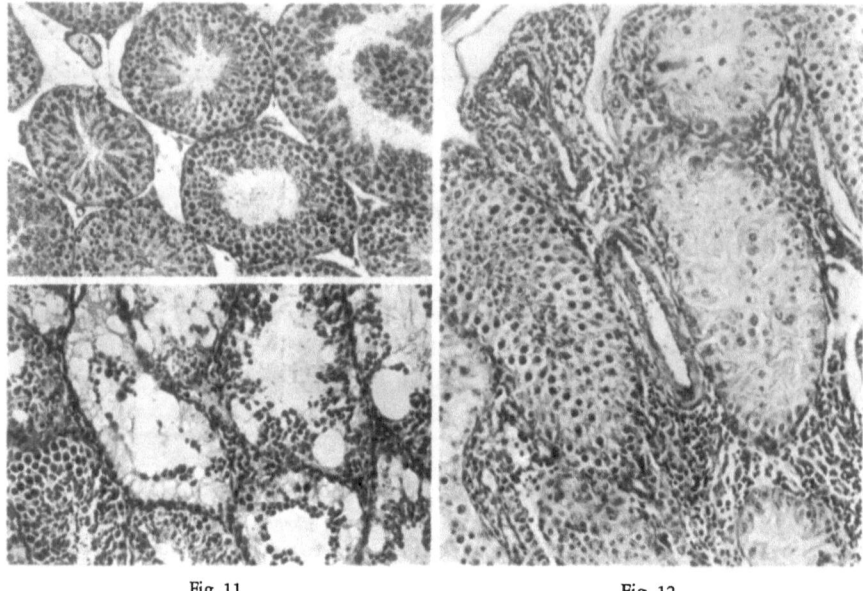

Fig. 11   Fig. 12

Fig. 11. *Top.* – Normal adult guinea pig testis. Seminiferous tubules with characteristic germinal epithelium; intertubular spaces showing small vessels and Leydig cells of normal appearance. *Bottom.* – An area of guinea pig testis 2 weeks after sensitization with testis homogenate in complete Freund's adjuvant. Seminiferous tubules displaying active sloughing and cytolysis of germinal cells. H & E. × 130

Fig. 12. Guinea pig testis 3 weeks after immunization with testis homogenate added with complete Freund's adjuvant. Seminiferous tubules showing different degree of sloughing and cytolysis of germinal cells. Perivascular and diffuse intertubular accumulation of mononuclear cells. H & E. × 140

germinative epithelium can be detected after the fourth month (BROWN *et al.,* 1956 and 1965). In another report (JOHNSON, 1970 a) animals were similarly sensitized and a booster dose was given two weeks later. Serial studies conducted from the 1st – 9th week revealed that damage is most readily observed in the rete testis and vasa efferentia but is less frequently present in the testis and epididymis. The testis shows interstitial inflammation and an invasion of tubules by eosinophils and mononuclear cells.

Histological observations of testes from guinea pigs, immunized with an ammonium sulphate precipitated fraction in complete adjuvant from 5 – 55 days, demonstrate that the pathologic picture varies depending upon the zone of examination. Most of the testes between 11 – 21 days exhibited monocytes and lymphocytes in the intertubular spaces, abutting against the tubular wall or even entering the lumen. Polymorphonuclear leukocytes were often prominent in severe lesions and observable either in the interstitium or inside the tubular lumen. After three weeks there were atrophic tubules surrounded by scanty inflammatory cells. During the sperm passage, lesions characterized by an acute exudate with polymorphonuclear cells were seen along the basement membrane of the ducts. In later lesions these cells entered the lumen and eventually

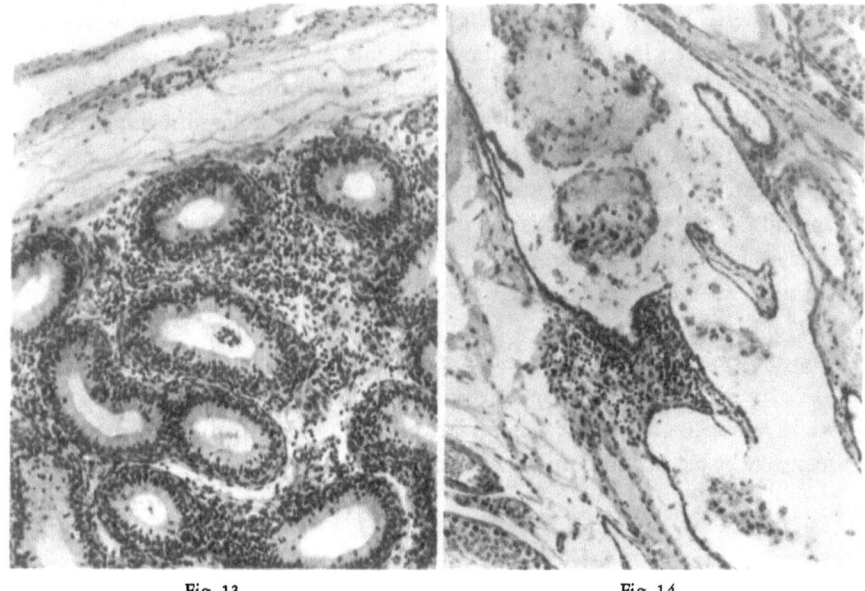

Fig. 13   Fig. 14

Fig. 13. Epididymis of guinea pig 3 weeks after immunization with testis homogenate added with complete Freund's adjuvant. Intercanalicular infiltration of mononuclear round cells. H & E. × 140

Fig. 14. Section of an area of the rete testis of guinea pig 4 weeks after immunization with testis homogenate plus complete Freund's adjuvant. Mononuclear cell accumulation in connective tissue subjacent to epithelium of the ducts. H & E. × 110

formed an abscess. In these cases a periductular accumulation of mononuclear cells was also found. These conditions were found in the straight tubules, rete testis, and the extratesticular structures, which include ductus efferens, epididymis, and vas deferens (TUNG et al., 1970).

As happens with induced antibodies when different antigens are used, the histological pattern of lesions may vary depending on the stimuli used. If, instead of autoclaved testis, papainized testis is used, intertubular infiltrations of cells are scanty. Moreover, when the autoclaved testis is treated with papain, the antigen is not destroyed, but the incidence of the lesion is lower and cell infiltration much less frequent (BROWN et al., 1963). It also seems that immunization with testicular homogenate or sperm cells, at variance with ammonium sulphate precipitated fraction, gives a more constant seminiferous tubule damage than inflammatory lesions in the rete testis and ductus efferens (TUNG et al., 1970).

The importance of using purified sperm antigens is reflected in experiments in which glycoprotein T, S, and P are injected together with complete adjuvant. The lesions are undistinguishable from each other at the mature stage, but early examination may show different primary lesions. Antigen T shows lesions characterized at the onset by aspermatogenesis, prior to significant cellular infiltration in the epididymis or in the

testis. In the testis lesions will appear later on. Antigen P induces lesions which begin
with cellular infiltrates in the head of the epididymis and in the rete testis. This cell accumulation appears in the epididymal tubules passing between parietal cells. Pseudo-
abscess formation and intense sclerosis may be seen later, as well as intense plasmocytic
accumulation. Testicular cell infiltration that follows an epididymal one is never polymorphonuclear but lymphomononuclear. Antigen S also provokes the appearance of
cellular infiltrates in the rete testis. In this case mononuclear accumulation, looking
like a delayed hypersensitive reaction, often predominates over polymorphonuclear infiltrate. In the testis the infiltration is always of the mononuclear type (VOISIN and TOUL-
LET, 1971).

From the preceding paragraphs it becomes clear why some authors who give priori-
ty to the germinal cell lesion have called this condition "autoimmune aspermatogenesis", while "autoallergic orchitis and epididymitis" has been used by those who consider the mesenchymal infiltration as the primary lesion.

b) Electron-Microscopy

With respect to the timing of sequential events leading to germinal epithelium lesions, a few studies at the electron-microscopic level have been made in immunized guinea pigs. It has been demonstrated that, from the 7th day onward after sensitization, dis-
crete ultrastructural changes appear to be developing in the region of the acrosomes; in
the late stages gross changes are found. Some of these early abnormalities are seldom
found in the testis of nonimmunized animals. The affected cells belong to early stages
of the maturation process of spermatids, and the later stages presumably have already
matured and left the seminiferous tubules; probably they have not been replaced as a
result of damage in the earlier stages (BROWN et al., 1972). The abnormalities evident
in the acrosomes of spermatids resemble those observed in these cells when incubated
in vitro with antisperm serum in the presence of complement (MANCINI et al., 1969; LE
BOUTELIER et al., 1973). According to recent observations (KIERSZENBAUM and MANCI-
NI, 1973), at the end of the 1st week there is moderate congestion and serous edema in
some intertubular areas, which coincides with the appearance of vacuolization of varying degree in the cytoplasm of Sertoli cells of neighbouring seminiferous tubules. During the 2nd and 3rd week vacuolization of Sertoli cells considerably increases. At the
same time, sloughing of germinal cells with clear signs of cytolysis has been observed
in an appreciable number of tubules, beginning with all types of spermatids and followed by spermatocytes (Figs. 15 – 16). Some of these cells showed eosinophilic cytoplasm or pycnotic nuclei. PAS positive acrosomes, detached from spermatids and masses
of fused acrosomes were also seen either near the sloughed cells, inside Sertoli cells
cytoplasm, or free in the lumen (MANCINI, 1964). The Sertoli cell cytoplasmic vesiculation appeared to stem from the distention of the smooth endoplasmic reticulum and
was followed by disruption and subsequent fusion of adjacent vesicles (Fig. 17). At the
onset, the retention of normal structure by the neighbouring germinal cells was in striking contrast to the changes in the Sertoli cells. After the 2nd week, when spermatids

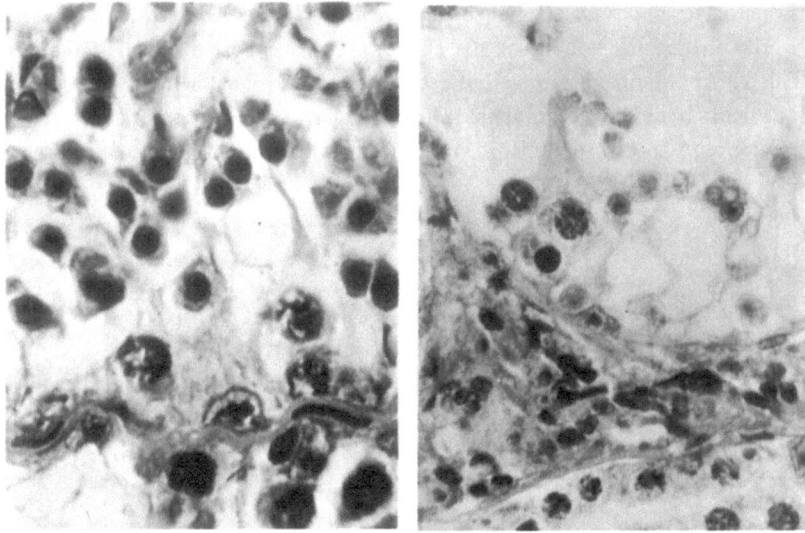

Fig. 15   Fig. 16

Fig. 15. Part of seminiferous tubule of guinea pig 1 week after sensitization with testis extract in complete adjuvant. Incipient vesiculation in the cytoplasm of a Sertoli cell. H & E. × 420. [KIERSZENBAUM and MANCINI; J. Reprod. Fertil. 33, 119 (1973)]

Fig. 16. Part of the seminiferous tubule of a guinea pig 4 weeks after sensitization. Advanced vesiculation of Sertoli cells and complete sloughing and cytolysis of spermatids and spermatocytes. Some spermatogonia are seen attached to internal part of tubular wall. H & E. × 420. [KIERSZENBAUM and MANCINI; J. Reprod. Fertil. 33, 119 (1973)]

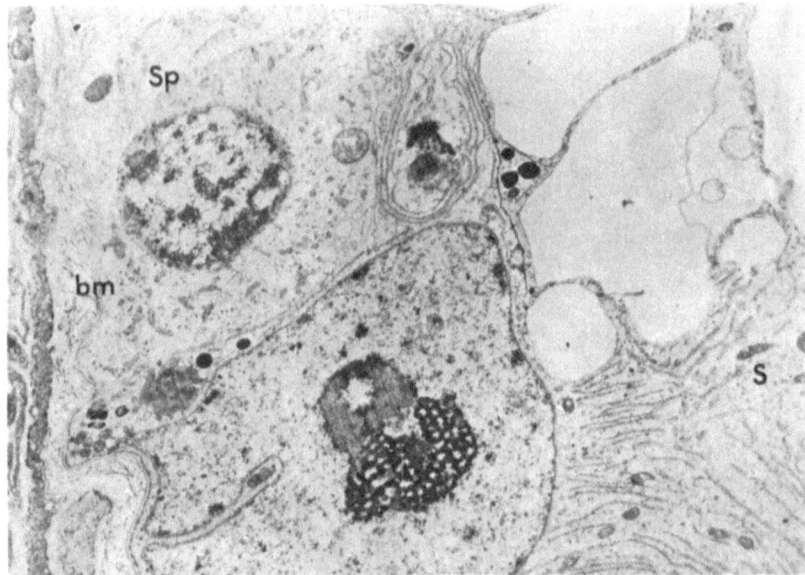

Fig. 17. A spermatogonia (Sp) and Sertoli cell (S) closely associated with the tubule wall; the cytoplasm of the Sertoli cell showing focal dilation of smooth endoplasmic reticulum cisternae in contrast to unchanged state of the spermatogonia. (bm: basement membrane). Electron-micrograph. × 9,000. [KIERSZENBAUM and MANCINI; J. Reprod. Fertil. 33, 119 (1973)]

and spermatocytes appeared affected by degenerative processes, Sertoli cells were en-
gaged in the phagocytosis of these cells, showing either engulfed cells or fragments of
cells. This enhanced phagocytic activity was closely associated with accumulation of
numerous dense bodies, lipid droplets, and different types of lysosomes (Figs. 18 – 19).
The appearance of an unusually large amount of chromatin clumps was prominent in

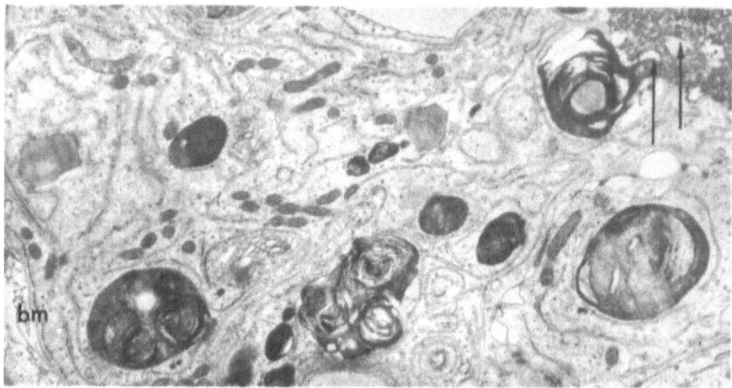

Fig. 18. A portion of cytoplasm of Sertoli cell showing a group of dense bodies, lipids droplets,
and lysosomes. The *arrow* points to a lysosome closely associated with debris of a phagocytosed
cell. (*bm:* basement membrane). Electron-micrograph. × 22,000. [KIERSZENBAUM and MANCINI;
J. Reprod. Fertil. 33, 119 (1973)]

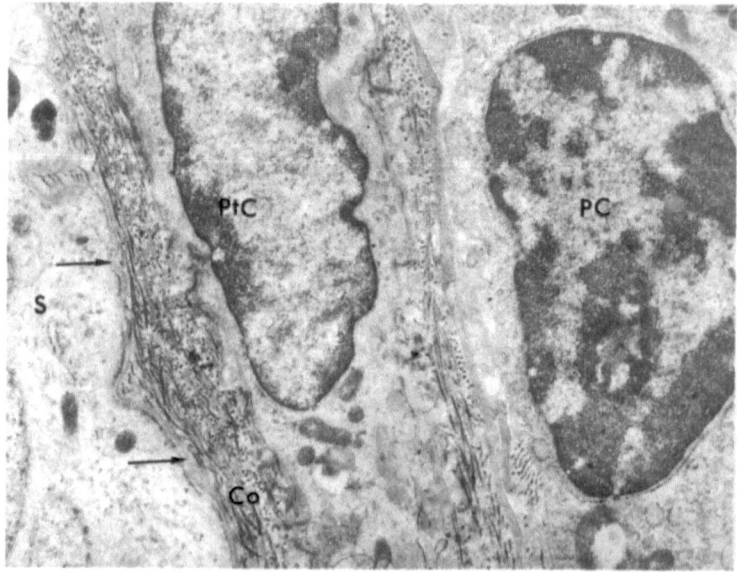

Fig. 19. Portion of a seminiferous tubule wall and boundary tissue. A plasma cell (*PC*) is shown
in close contact with collagen fibers (*Co*) and with peritubular cell (*PtC*). The unchanged state
of the different components of the seminiferous tubular wall, especially the basement membrane
(*arrow*) can be seen (*S:* Sertoli cell). Electron-micrograph. × 26,000 [KIERSZENBAUM and MANCI-
NI; J. Reprod. Fertil. 33, 119 (1973)]

some nuclei. Whether or not these modifications of the nuclear structure were related to increased phagocytic activity is uncertain. No changes could be observed in the mitochondria and Golgi apparatus nor in any other cytoplasmic areas of Sertoli cells, where rough reticuloendoplasmic cisternae displayed normal features. Although nuclear pycnosis or cytolysis was common in germinal cells, other anomalies occurring in spermatids were indicated by coarse chromatin, accumulations of granular material in nuclei (interchromatin granules), and extensive attachment of granules, probably ribosomes, to the acrosomal cap.

In the intertubular spaces, perivascular infiltration of mononuclear cells interpersed with scattered polymorphonuclear leukocytes increased and some small and medium-sized arterioles showed hyperplastic and hypertrophic endothelium. The internal portion of the seminiferous tubule walls adjacent to Sertoli cells was not seen in intimate contact with inflammatory cells. Neither was the transit of those cells into the seminiferous tubules through defects in the basal lamina observed. However, the erratic presence of plasmocytes or lymphocytes close to the tubular wall and inside the tubule in contact with germinal cells was detected (Fig. 19). The ultrastructural feature of the basal lamina, subjacent network of collagen fibrils and layers of peritubular cells disclosed no obvious modifications in the presence of extensive peritubular infiltration. From the 4th – 6th week the majority of the seminiferous tubules contained no germinal cells. Some of them still had a few spermatogonial cells showing apparently normal ultrastructural features. Sertoli cells with intact nuclei and nucleoli showed a hypertrophied cytoplasm filled with large vacuoles, and debris of membranous material remained in the tubules. In the intertubular spaces a low number of mononuclear cells were still identifiable (KIERSZENBAUM and MANCINI, 1973).

It can be concluded that in the early stages of postimmunization there was a constant vesiculation in Sertoli cell cytoplasm, which is either preceded or accompanied by germinal cells cytolysis and sloughing. This phenomenon is characterized by vascular changes in the intertubular spaces. Existing evidence strongly suggests that lesions are primarily apparent in the Sertoli cells and spermatids, but that the damage and sloughing of spermatocytes and spermatogonial cells in the sequence of events requires further study.

7. Pathogenesis

In general, immunopathologic lesions may arise from hypersensitivity reactions or from immunotoxic interaction. The contact of the sensitizing agent with the corresponding humoral antibody or sensitized cell constitutes a trigger mechanism which may activate the complement system and probably induces the release of mediators such as histamines, serotonin, or bradykinin-like substances. As a result, increased permeability, edema, chemotaxis of leukocytes, and tissue necrosis take place in the host tissue. On the other hand, the formation of a macromolecular aggregate of the immune complex type may act as a foreign body, thus attracting leukocytes or causing disturbances in the nutrition of the tissue. Interaction between antibodies and sensitized cells may produce a synergistic or antagonistic effect. The possibility of this interaction depends on the accessibility of the target cell to the immune agent, which in turn depends on the vascular and tissue permeability. As regards the mechanism of the production of allergic orchitis, there is no agreement yet about the role of cellular immunity or of the different humoral antibodies in this characteristic immunotoxic reaction.

a) Morphologic Basis

Since the early description of this experimental disease, it was concluded that the autoallergic lesion of the testis was mainly due to sensitivity to the delayed or tuberculin type of reaction. This was based on: (1) the presence of mycobacteria in the antigenic mixture used, (2) the effectiveness of the intradermal route of inoculation, (3) the poor correlation of the process with humoral antibodies and (4) the clearly established presence of skin reactivity to testis antigen and the positivity of macrophage migration inhibition test. Delayed reaction consists of foci of perivenous inflammation; lymphocytes and histiocytes are the principal reacting cells and parenchymal damage occurs only in cases of intense reactions. The similarity between this histological picture and that described in the testis is obvious. In addition, when tubercle bacilli or tuberculin are injected into the testis of a tuberculin sensitive guinea pig, the resulting lesion is comparable to that of allergic orchitis (WAKSMAN, 1959 a). There are other experimental immunologic diseases, such as allergic encephalomyelitis, where the initial lesion also appears as an irregularly disseminated focal inflammatory disease and in which parenchymal destruction is associated with invasion of the nervous tissue by mononuclear cells. This disease is also poorly correlated with humoral antibody. It is interesting to note that nonimmunologic destruction of myelin fails to produce inflammation comparable to that seen in the experimental disease. The final disappearance of germinal cells should therefore be regarded as a result of a nonspecific secondary disturbance due to swelling and circulatory interference (WAKSMAN, 1959 b).

Inflammatory edema, increased tissue pressure, ischemia, and sometimes infarction have been described in immunized rats, giving support to the concept of allergic orchitis rather than allergic aspermatogenesis (LEVINE and SOWINSKY, 1970). Furthermore, a polypeptide probably related to bradykinin, as deduced from its biological action upon smooth muscle and the lytic effect of chymotrypsin, is present in testicular extracts of guinea pigs soon after sensitization. It would be premature to state that this vasoactive substance plays a definite role in the testicular allergic inflammation, but it is interesting to point out that its higher concentration in the gonad coincides with the early development of congestion and serous edema in the intertubular spaces (MANCINI et al., 1966) (Table 4).

Table 4. Correlation between amount of polypeptide in testicular tissue and percentage of animals showing release of polypeptide, testicular lesion, and circulating antibody in each period, after sensitization of guinea pigs with testis homogenate mixed with complete Freund's adjuvant. [MANCINI, HUIDOBRO, F. COLLAZO, and MONASTIRSKY; Proc. Soc. Exp. Biol. Med. 123, 227 (1966)]

			% of animals showing		
Days after sensitization	No. of animals	Amt of polypeptide in testicular tissue ($\mu g/g$)	Polypeptide in testicular tissue	Testicular lesion	Circulating antibody
3– 5	12	$.38 \pm .11$ (p .05)	58.3	33.3	25.0
23–26	14	$1.23 \pm .21$ (p .05)	100.0	78.6	50.0
12–15	12	$1.03 \pm .22$ (p .05)	83.3	75.0	33.3
36–40	11	$.40 \pm .08$	100.0	72.7	45.4

b) Role of Humoral Antibodies

Although humoral antisperm antibodies can be demonstrated in sensitized animals and their cytotoxicity upon spermatozoa and spermatids has been observed *in vitro* (MANCINI et al., 1969; LE BOUTELIER et al., 1973), there are facts that militate against their participation in the tubule damage, namely: (a) Repeated injections during several weeks or months of homologous serum containing antibody detectable by serologic and/or biological techniques fail to transmit the disease. (b) There is no strict correlation between histological lesions of the testis and the presence of these antibodies (FREUND et al., 1953, BISHOP and CARLSON, 1965; BROWN et al., 1967). Nevertheless, aspermatogenesis has been consistently produced when the recipient guinea pig was intradermally pretreated with Freund's complete adjuvant alone, 7 days prior to transfer of serum from a donor homologous animal which was itself immunized previously

with testicular homogenate in complete Freund's adjuvant. It was postulated that the
adjuvant modifies in some manner the recipient animal, so that the antibody can gain
access to the seminiferous epithelium by affecting the tubular barrier (POKORNA, 1970;
WILSON et al., 1972). More detailed, recent studies have shown that antisperm humoral
antibodies, when injected into normal guinea pigs either systemically or into the interstitium of the testis, bind the sperm inside the rete testis and produce a mild acute inflammatory reaction at that site. I–125 labeled IgG from normal guinea pigs, when injected into the testis, can cross the wall of the rete testis and enter into the lumen. The
serum proteins, on the other hand, do not appear to penetrate the seminiferous tubules.
These results suggest that an antibody, although not directly involved in the production of aspermatogenesis, can produce an acute inflammatory reaction by binding
sperm in the sperm passage system (TUNG et al., 1971 a). In this report, observations
have only been made during the 1st week after the local injection, but further studies
using similar methodology and a more prolonged period of examination (MANCINI
et al., 1974) suggest that not only rete testis lesions develop but that damage of tubular
germinal cells, accompanied by intertubular accumulation of mononuclear cells, may
be detected within the 3rd – 7th week. In the 1st week a transient polymorphonuclear
infiltration occurs in the interstitium. These results, which do not imply a direct action
of antibodies on seminiferous tubules, show that after the induction of an inflammation of the rete testis and vasa efferentia, antisperm serum locally injected can evoke,
through an as yet unknown mechanism, focal lesions of allergic orchitis.

The importance and significance of rete testis and vasa efferentia in the histogenesis
of allergic orchitis has been substantiated recently (JOHNSON, 1970 b). The greater vul-
nerability of these structures is understandable, because the blood barrier of the rete testis in normal conditions is less effective than that of seminiferous tubules to serum
proteins (MANCINI et al., 1965; KORMANO, 1968). Phagocytosis of sperm by intratubular macrophages also occurs in this part of the tract (RISLEY, 1963). There is a slight increase in the permeability of the seminiferous tubules to the fluorescent dye acroflavin,
soon after isoimmunization of guinea pigs. The permeability increase might initially be
due to a spread of interstitial inflammation from the rete, thus allowing entry of humoral and cellular immunity antibodies. Alternately, following entry of a small
amount of antibody, release of acrosomal enzymes could make the tubule leaky. Thus,
induction of testicular damage may be seen as dependent upon the immune response
of whatever type, overcoming the resistance presented by the tubular barrier. This assumption has been reinforced by the fact that immune lesions develop in only a few
puberal animals after sensitization, in which spermatozoal antigen had not yet entered
the rete testis. The incidence is raised after experimental weakening of the blood testis
barrier with cadmium or by an induced traumatisation or inflammation of the gland
(JOHNSON, 1970 a, b).

Favoring the assumption that humoral antibodies may participate in the development of tubule lesions is the hypothesis (KARUSH and EISEN, 1962) that delayed hypersensitivity is not due to sensitized cells, but is the result of a reaction to a special type
of antibody, produced in amounts not detectable by ordinary immunological methods,
but capable of producing skin reactions because of avidity for antigen. If such an anti-

body were responsible for the testicular damage, it would explain the absence of infil-
trating cells in the early stages of the testes lesions in guinea pigs sensitized with papainized testicular material. Thus, the essential antigen present in this material responsible
for the lesion fails to produce a positive skin test in animals immunized with whole testis. Accordingly, if these lesions are due to some form of delayed hypersensitivity, it
must be assumed that the factors responsible are entirely removed from the circulation
by the testis (BROWN et al., 1963).

c) Role of Cellular Immunity

The development of testis lesion in animals which do not show positive skin reaction makes it difficult to reconcile this phenomena with the generally accepted hypothesis that this damage is directly mediated by specifically sensitized cells of the kind responsible for skin reaction. However, the possibility of transferring this disease to secondary recipients by means of sensitized mononuclear cells has recently been demonstrated. Following the successful transfer in guinea pigs of delayed cutaneous sensitivity
with lymph node cells from homologous testes-immunized donor animals (BOUGHTON
and SCHILD, 1962), the induction of typical testicular lesions, using cells from peritoneal exudate or from lymph node in inbred rats (LAURENCE et al., 1965) and guinea pigs
(STONE et al., 1969) has been reported. Intratesticular transfer of cells extracted from
lymph nodes of homologous guinea pigs, 5 – 7 days after immunization with testicular
antigens administered with complete adjuvant, also resulted in the formation of an extensive intertubular granuloma composed of lymphocytes, plasmocytes and macrophages. This condition, which developed 6 – 14 days after intratesticular injection, was accompanied by destruction of germinal cells, persistence of Sertoli and Leydig cells and
the penetration of some mononuclear cells into the seminiferous tubules (MANCINI,
1968 a). Recently, the experimental allergic orchitis has been passively transferred in
histocompatible guinea pigs by lymph node cells from animals immunized with sperm
in complete Freund's adjuvant. Systemic injection of sensitized cells produces at best
mild lesions in the recipients. However, local transfer of cells into the interstitium of
the testis initiated severe changes within 4 – 8 days. The lesion was identical to that
observed in the primary disease, and characterized by an intertubular infiltration of
monocytes that preceded degeneration of the germinal epithelium. The monocytes
and macrophages were of host origin and their precursors were radiosensitive. The
lymph node cells had to be alive and removed from a guinea pig immune to sperm and
not to other tissue or organs. The characteristics of the lesion, the lack of infiltration of
neutrophils, the absence of detectable antibody bound to sperm in the tubules and
sperm passage system and the rapidity with which the lesion develops are strong evidence that antisperm antibody, if formed, participates only to a small extent in the
tubular damage. The interpretation of these results is that mononuclear cells involved
in the process come from the blood and must penetrate the seminiferous tubules in
order to react with germinal cells by an unknown mechanism (TUNG et al., 1971 b).

Experimental allergic orchitis was also transferred to the same strain of guinea pigs by the intratesticular injection of sensitized peritoneal exudate cells obtained from syngeneic donors immunized with a testicular antigen in complete Freund's adjuvant (KANTOR and DIXON, 1972). The lesions obtained were typical of this experimental disease, antigen and organ specific; they developed within 24 hrs of transfer, and consisted of macrophages and polymorphonuclear leukocytes within the seminiferous tubules, rete testis and, interstitial tissue, leading finally to aspermatogenesis. By immunofluorescence neither gamma-globulin nor complement were detectable within the edematous areas of the interstitium. When contrasted with the behaviour of lymph nodes, sensitized peritoneal cell exudate induces lesions sooner and more frequently, and requires fewer total cells and lymphocytes per transfer, resulting in a more intense infiltrative process particularly in the rete testis. The recruitment of mononuclear and phagocytic effector cells from the recipient is also essential since the resultant lesions may be prevented by irradiation of the host just prior to cell transfer. Presumably the local transfer of peritoneal exudate cells, containing both sensitized lymphocytes and activated macrophages, results in the production of an early and intense lesion. Moreover, an RNA preparation extracted from lymph nodes or spleen of guinea pigs sensitized with testis plus added adjuvant is capable of passively transferring the immunologic orchitis to homologous normal animals (FAINBOIM et al., 1975).

In spite of the strong evidence in favour of the participation of delayed hypersensitivity or cellular immunity in the pathogenesis of immune orchitis, the contention that mononuclear cell infiltration in the testis is a secondary phenomenon and the fact that testicular lesions may be present in animals not showing delayed skin reaction make it difficult to accept the hypothesis that the tubular lesion is directly and primarily mediated by specifically sensitized cells of the kind responsible for skin reaction.

d) Requirement for Both Antibodies

A new hypothesis on the dual necessity for both antibodies, in humoral and cellular immunity, has been advanced (BROWN et al., 1967). Experiments to substantiate this theory were set up as follows: (1) Guinea pigs injected with testis homogenate plus incomplete adjuvant developed antibodies but no delayed hypersensitivity or testicular lesions. These animals failed to show delayed hypersensitivity or testis lesion when subsequently injected with antigen in complete adjuvant. Animals similarly treated and then given repeated injections of lymph node immune cells from animals immunized with whole testis and complete adjuvant developed both delayed skin reaction and the characteristic orchitis. (2) Animals sensitized with a purified testicular glycoprotein preparation in complete adjuvant developed delayed hypersensitivity but had no circulating antibodies or testicular lesion. When repeated injections of homologous serum containing antitestis antibody were given, some of the animals developed orchitis. (3) A study of animals killed at daily intervals after injection with testicular antigen plus complete adjuvant showed that an antibody was detectable by immunofluorescence inside the seminiferous tubules on the same day as delayed hypersensitivity appeared. Humoral antibody was not detected until two days later. In addition, antibody was not detectable in the testes in any animal in the absence of delayed hypersensitivity.

These experiments led the authors to the conclusion that delayed hypersensitivity or humoral antibody alone are not sufficient to produce testicular lesions. Immunized animals which fail to give a delayed skin reaction after receiving immune cells are contrasted with guinea pigs which showed circulating antibody after receiving the same cells, but did give a positive reaction. This behavior is in line with earlier statements that circulating antibodies potentiate the delayed hypersensitivity (ASHERSON and LOEWI, 1966). The fact that antibody is demonstrable within the seminiferous tubules on the same day as delayed hypersensitivity suggests that the presence of antibody in the tubules, in spite of the absence of peritubular cell infiltration, is dependent upon the presence of delayed hypersensitivity. The fact that humoral antibody is not detectable two to four days later may be explained by the low titer in the serum in the early stages or a high avidity for germinal cells associated with delayed hypersensitivity (KARUSH and EISEN, 1962). This is supported by the situation described in sheep nephritis, where the absence of antibody in the serum is attributable to uptake of antibody by antigen in the involved organ (LERNER and DIXON, 1966).

The need for both types of immunologic reaction is reinforced by other experiments in which purified guinea pig spermatozoal antigens were used (TOULLET and VOISIN, 1969). The chronologic and quantitative appearance of three types of hypersensitivity, that is anaphylactic, Arthus and delayed, as well as the state of vascular permeability in the testis and the degree of damage in the germinal epithelium, were examined. It was seen that there was a significant correlation between seminiferous tubule lesions, the simultaneous presence of both delayed and anaphylactic types of hypersensitivity and an increase in the vascular and tissue permeability in the epididymis, rete testis, and testicular structures. The enhanced permeability is considered highly significant and is probably induced by cellular immunity mediators to make the target tissues accessible to active antibodies.

As regards the vascular phenomena, it has been reported that histamine, acetylcholine, and serotonin were not detectable in the testicular tissue of guinea pigs after sensitization with testis applied with complete adjuvant. However, as mentioned before, a polypeptide substance related to bradykinin was present in an higher amount during the first few weeks and began to disappear around the fourth week. A close correlation was also noted between the appearance of this polypeptide and the edema occurring in the intertubular spaces during the first days preceding inflammation and signs of germinal cell lesions (MANCINI et al., 1966). Several peptides like bradykinin and related substances have been found in different tissues and their action is sufficiently potent to suggest that their function might result in increased permeability and migration of blood cells. Further studies are required to clarify the bradykinin forming mechanism and its correlation with antigen-antibody interaction in allergic orchitis.

e) Role of Sertoli Cells

Regarding the role of Sertoli cells in the immunologic mechanism of sloughing and cytolysis of germinal cells, it must be borne in mind that all of these cells, except spermatogonia, are normally in close contact with the cytoplasm of Sertoli cells. Secondly, the concept of the supportive and nutritional function of these cells has been reinforced by experiments showing that the intratubular penetration of a variety of circulating substances, including proteins, may take place through the cytoplasm and intercellular spaces which separate Sertoli cells from the germinal ones (MANCINI et al., 1965; FAWCETT et al., 1970). Consequently, it is possible to assume that antisperm antibodies, whether circulating and/or mononuclear cell mediated, may gain access and interact with antigenic germinal cells by way of Sertoli cell cytoplasm or through intercellular spaces. The marked dilatation of the reticulum endoplasmic cisternae described above may reflect an early sign of the response of the Sertoli cells to the immunogenic injury. The progressive vacuolation could impair the Sertoli-germinal cell relationship, with subsequent sloughing of the germinal elements. Detachment of germinal cells may be facilitated by the marginal vacuoles present in Sertoli cell cytoplasm and not by a direct disruption of intercellular bindings. At the same time, direct interaction of antibodies with germinal cells could take place and cytolysis would develop (KIERSZENBAUM and MANCINI, 1973). This interpretation appears to be supported by the fact that labeled antisperm antibodies react with the acrosome of spermatids and spermatozoa, and not with Sertoli cell cytoplasm. All these events represent perhaps a nonspecific reaction of Sertoli cells to several types of aggression, for they are also observed in animals treated with cytostatic drugs or in the postirradiation period, that is under conditions which also cause vacuolization of Sertoli cells, sloughing and necrobiosis of germinal cells.

f) Relation to Homograft Rejection

Allergic orchitis and homograft rejection share certain common characteristics, but a delayed type of immune response is involved in both systems. The antigens identified in both conditions seem to be polypeptide-polysaccharide complexes; another similarity resides in the localization of autoantigens and histocompatible testicular antigens in the acrosome of sperm cells (VÓJTISKOVÁ and POKORNÁ, 1971; ERICKSON, 1971). However, allergic aspermatogenesis implies cell deterioration of the host testis and is provoked by the injection of either whole testis homogenate, extracts of spermatic cells or selective antigens, whereas the homograft reaction leads to destruction of implanted tissue which has been introduced as intact organ with living cells. These phenomena which undoubtedly deserve further study have been regarded as the mutual incompatibility of autoantigens and homograft antigens present in a given tissue (VOISIN et al., 1958; BISHOP et al., 1961). Studies of homotransplantation of the whole testis with vascular anastomosis have been made in noninbred dogs (ATTARAN et al., 1966) and in inbred rats (LEE et al., 1971). With respect to transplants of the gonad in adult nonhisto-

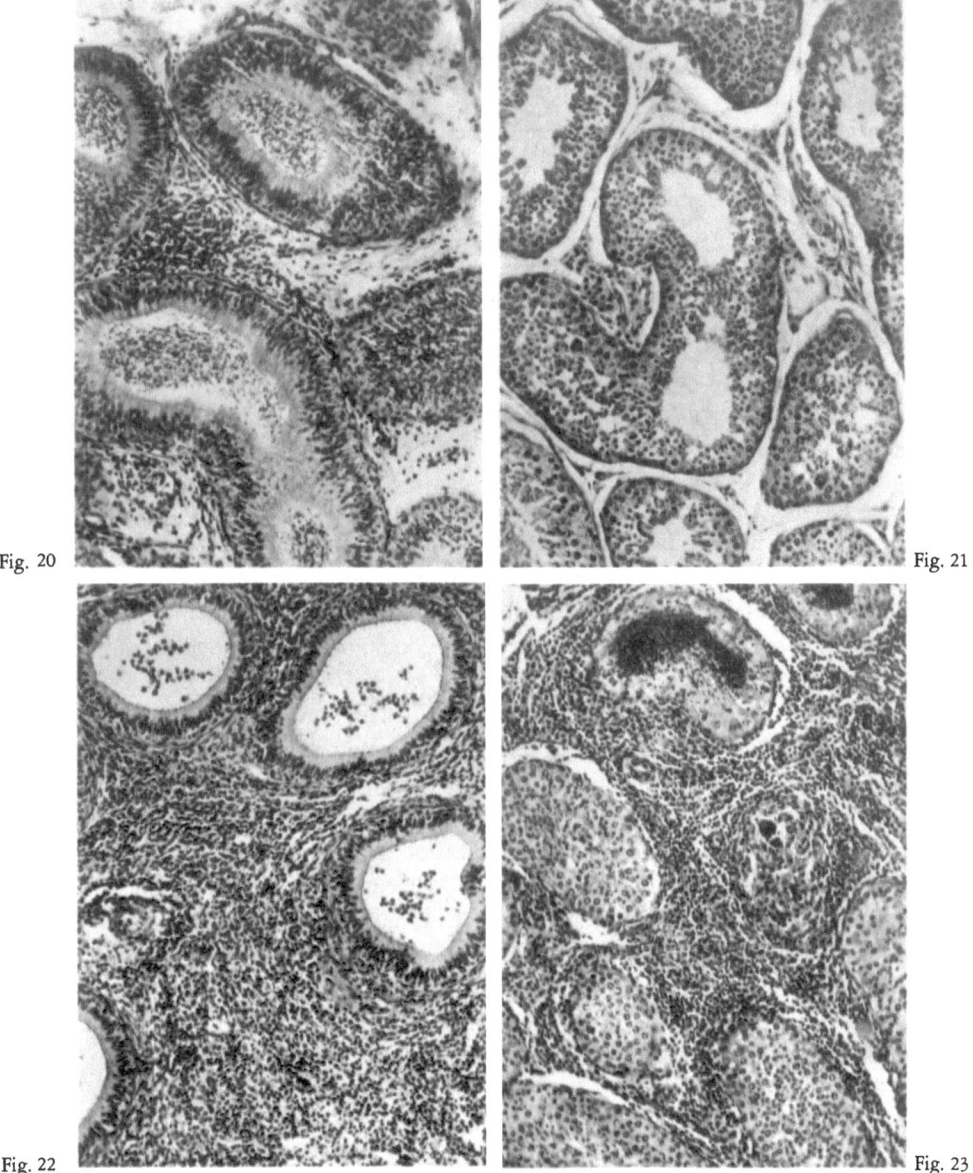

Fig. 20
Fig. 21
Fig. 22
Fig. 23

Fig. 20. Testis of dog 4 days after homotransplantation. Mononuclear cell infiltration in intercanalicular spaces of epididymis. The epithelium appears normal and clumps of spermatozoa are present in the lumen. H & E. × 140. [MANCINI, GALLO MORANDO, TORRES and PAHUL; Medicina 32, 215 (1972)]

Fig. 21. Same as in Fig. 20. Seminiferous tubules displaying some areas of slight sloughing of germinal cells. Leydig cells and vessels in the intertubular spaces with normal appearance. H & E. × 140 [MANCINI et al.; Medicina 32, 215 (1972)]

Fig.22. Testis of a dog 7 days after homologous transplantation. Intense and diffuse mononuclear cell infiltration in the intercanalicular spaces of epididymis. No spermatozoa but germinal cells are present in the lumen. H & E. × 140 [MANCINI et al.; Medicina 32, 215 (1972)]

Fig. 23. Same as in Fig. 22. Seminiferous tubules showing partially atrophied germinal epithelium are surrounded by a dense accumulation of mononuclear cells. Some small groups of Leydig cells are still identifiable. H & E. × 140 [MANCINI et al.; Medicina 32, 215 (1972)]

compatible dogs, the sequential histological study of the rejection phenomenon, which takes place around the sixth day, indicated that mononuclear cells invade the tissue in a manner encountered in allergic aspermatogenesis. Infiltration begins in the intercanalicular spaces of the epididymis, extends into the albuginea and septa of the gonad and then spreads around the rete testis and seminiferous tubules (Figs. 20 – 23). Later on and coinciding with cytolysis of germinal cells, lymphocytes and plasmocytes appear inside the tubules within the germinative epithelium (MANCINI et al., 1972). No data are available on the development of humoral antisperm antibodies or cellular immunity, as established in experimental allergic orchitis.

g) Sensitization in the Absence of Adjuvants

The role of complete Freund's adjuvant has repeatedly been discussed in the mechanism of the production of allergic orchitis, not only because of its potentiating ability of antigens and formation of a dermal granuloma, but also in connection with the induction of cellular immunity. Incomplete Freund's adjuvant induces only the anaphylactic type of antibodies (local or systemic); it does not induce testicular lesion, delayed hypersensitivity, or fixing complement and precipitating antibodies. It has been claimed that repeated injections of homologous testicular homogenate alone for several months apparently provoke mild focal lesions of aspermatogenesis in guinea pigs, but antibodies have been completely unexplored (BISHOP, 1961). In an attempt to induce lesions in the contralateral gland of guinea pigs, one testis was interstitially injected with turpentine while complete Freund's adjuvant was administered subcutaneously (BOUGHTON and SPECTOR, 1963); in another experiment, a unilateral intratesticular injection of complete Freund's adjuvant was given to rats, guinea pigs, and rabbits (EYQUEM and KRIEG, 1965). In both cases mild foci of allergic orchitis developed in the contralateral testis and some positive results were observed with the immunoserologic techniques used. A model describing circulating antibodies and lesions in the contralateral testis after unilateral thermal orchitis in guinea pigs has been described some time ago (RAPAPPORT et al., 1969). In this report no attention was paid to delayed hypersensitivity, epididymal lesion, or the possible potentiating effect of added Freund's adjuvant. Therefore, a series of experiments has been performed in order to verify the need for adjuvants in sperm sensitization (Table 5).

Effect of Unilateral Thermal Orchitis on the Contralateral Gonad. The effect of endogenous sensitization of guinea pigs by products deriving from thermal orchitis with or without the addition of complete Freund's adjuvant was examined. For this purpose, unilateral thermal orchitis (left testis) was induced under general anaesthesia in a group of adult guinea pigs by intratesticular instillation with 1ml of boiling saline. In another group this was followed by intradermal injection of 0.5 ml of complete Freund's adjuvant in the left thigh. The immunologic response and lesions which developed in the contralateral gland were serially studied from 1 – 8 weeks. It was found that (1) with the exception of the sperm immobilizing test, which was positive in some animals, no detectable antisperm antibodies of complement fixing or precipitating

Table 5. *From Top to Bottom. Different Groups of Experiments. First Group.* Correlation among type of adjuvant used in homologous systemic sensitization procedure, immunologic response, and testis lesion.
Second Group. Lesion in the contralateral gonad and antibodies, developed in response to unilateral damage of testis induced with various types of inflammatory injury.
Third Group. Damage in the contralateral gonad and antibodies, developed as a consequence of thermal or traumatic injury in the opposite gonad. Immunogenic potency of homogenates prepared with these abnormal testes in homologous sensitization are also listed.

Abbreviations
C-F: Complement fixing test
P.C.A.: Passive cutaneous anaphylaxis
I.M.M.: Inhibition monophage migration

Group	Antigenic stimuli	Complete or incomplete Freund's adjuvant	Site of injection	Immunological response					Testicular response
				Humoral antibodies		Cellular immunity			
1	Normal testicular homogenate	Complete	Subcutaneous (single dose)	Precipit. C-F immov. agglutin. P.C.A. anafilac.	+ + + + + +	Skin test. I.M.M.	+ +		Diffuse allergic orchitis
	Normal testicular homogenate	Incomplete	Subcutaneous (single dose)	Immov. P.C.A. anafilac.	+ + +	Skin test. I.M.M.	– –		No damage
	Normal testicular homogenate	None	Subcutaneous (many doses)	P.C.A.	+	Not done			Multifocal allergic orchitis
2	None	Complete	Subcutaneous plus turpentine intratesticular (unilateral)	Not done		Not done			Focal allergic orchitis (contralateral gland)
	None	None	Turpentine intratesticular (unilateral)	Not done		Not done			No damage (contralateral gland)
	None	Complete	Intratesticular (unilateral)	C-F hemaggl. P.C.A.	+ + +	Skin test.	+		Multifocal allergic orchitis (Same gland)

Pathogenesis

Table 5 (continued)

Group	Antigenic stimuli	Complete or incomplete Freund's adjuvant	Site of injection	Immunological response		
				Humoral antibodies	Cellular immunity	Testicular response
3	None	None	Thermal injury (unilateral)	C-F precipit. − precipit. + immov. + P.C.A. +	− Skin test.	+ Multifocal allergic orchitis (contralat. gland)
	Homogenate from thermal injured testis	None	Subcutaneous (single dose) (homologous)	Precipit. − C-F − immov. + P.C.A. +	− Skin test. − I.M.M.	+ Multifocal allergic orchitis (Both glands)
	None	None	Traumatic injury (unilateral)	Precipit. − hemaggl. − agglutin. + P.C.A. +	− Skin test. − I.M.M.	+ Multifocal allergic orchitis (contralat. gland)

types appeared. (2) Delayed hypersensitivity as revealed by skin test, and inhibition of macrophage migration was positive. (3) While in the injured testis an acute inflammation followed by a granulomatous reaction developed during the first few weeks, lesions resembling those of allergic orchitis appeared in the contralateral gonad and epididymis. (4) No difference was detectable in this immunologic response when the injured animals were in addition injected with complete Freund's adjuvant (FERNÁNDEZ COLLAZO et al., 1972).

These results indicate that severe heat damage in one testis may be followed by lesions typical of the so-called allergic orchitis in the contralateral organ, accompanied by an immunologic response of the delayed type as revealed by skin test (Figs. 24 – 27). These findings corroborate and amplify those reported on the same subject (RAPPAPORT et al., 1969). The absence of circulating antisperm antibodies of complement-fixing type has also been confirmed. The positive skin test and contralateral testis-epididymal lesions in the advanced stage of these experiments recall findings encountered in the classical allergic orchitis. As these lesions developed during the 2nd and 3rd week after injury, a higher correlation with delayed hypersensitivity and the intertubular granulomatous reaction than with circulating antibodies seems likely. Evidently, thermal injury to the guinea pig testis, at variance with the classical induced allergic

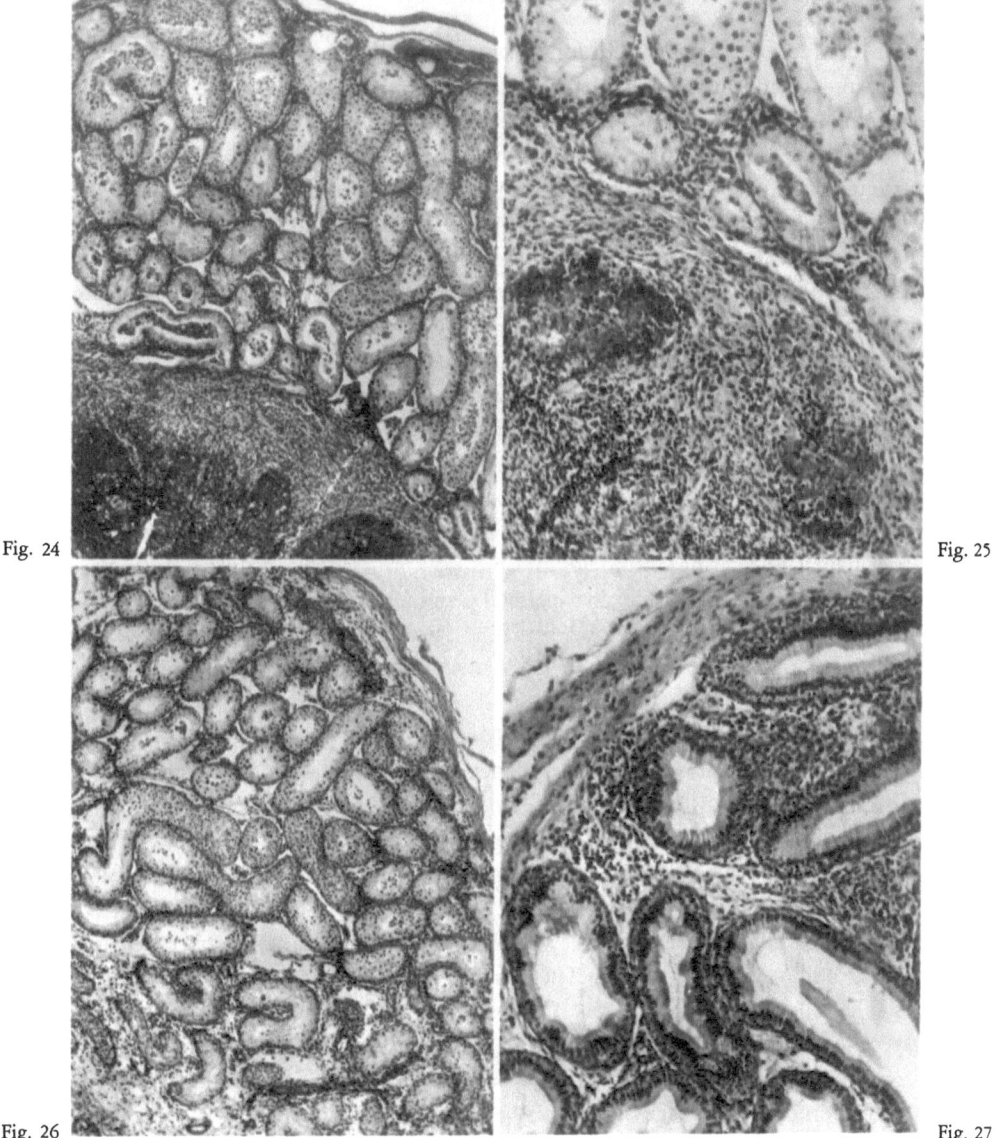

Fig. 24. Guinea pig left testis 3 days after thermal injury. A central necrotic area surrounded by an inflammatory zone and a cortical one with seminiferous tubules showing sloughed germinal cells. H & E. × 80 [FERNÁNDEZ COLLAZO, THIERER, and MANCINI; J. Allergy and Clin. Immunol. 49, 167 (1972)]

Fig. 25. Same as in Fig. 24 at higher magnification; the inflammatory area displaying a granulomatous reaction of histiocytes, mononuclear cells, and macrophages. H & E. × 220 [FERNÁNDEZ COLLAZO et al.; J. Allergy and Clin. Immunol. 49, 167 (1972)]

Fig. 26. Contralateral right testis of same guinea pig 21 days after thermal injury in left testis. Multifocal lesions of allergic orchitis. Seminiferous tubules with cytolisis of germinal cells and intertubular accumulation of mononuclear cells, also seen behind the tunica albuginea. H & E. × 80 [FERNÁNDEZ COLLAZO et al.; J. Allergy and Clin. Immunol. 49, 167 (1972)]

Fig. 27. Epididymis of contralateral testis showing infiltration of mononuclear cells in intercanalicular spaces. Spermatozoa together with germinal cells are also present in the lumen. H & E. × 80 [FERNÁNDEZ COLLAZO et al.; J. Allergy and Clin. Immunol. 49, 167 (1972)]

orchitis, does not require the addition of adjuvant and can evoke a similar response. On the other hand, the need for the simultaneous presence of destroyed germinal epithelium and Freund's adjuvant in the production of unilateral orchitis has been substantiated by the induction of a local inflammation in the contralateral testis in response to an intradermal injection of the adjuvant or by the injection into the contralateral testis of the adjuvant alone. It is emphasized that only fairly extensive lesions in the injected left testis are concomitant with the development of lesions in the contralateral gland. The only possible source of spermatic "autoantigens" in this phenomenon seems to be the thermally injured testis. The question therefore arises as to whether the necrotic, inflammatory, or cortical subnormal area is liberating or producing abnormal proteins capable of behaving as antigen, which in turn induces the local intratesticular granuloma. In connection with the damaging effect of extreme variations in temperature it has been demonstrated that antibodies against a given tissue may also be elicited by freezing that organ *in situ* (SHULMAN *et al.,* 1967). Furthermore, repeated *in situ* freezing of a liquid nitrogen cooled probe has been shown to result in the formation of circulating hemagglutinating antibodies and probably in changes occurring not only in the injured gonad but also in the contralateral gland (ABLIN *et al.,* 1971). Detailed studies have been made in rabbits, showing that 1 – 4 weeks after cryo-injury of the right testis, striking changes in the content of ductus epididymidis and in seminiferous tubules of the left testis appeared, and these changes were regarded as an expression of an autoallergic reaction (ZAPPI and SHULMAN, 1974).

Homologous Sensitization with Thermal Orchitis Homogenate. In conjunction with the above results it was considered desirable to verify the antigenic potency of homogenates prepared from heat-damaged guinea pig testis in homologous sensitization. Adult outbred guinea pigs were sensitized (without adjuvant) with a single dose of homogenate, prepared from homologous testis, that had been previously subjected *in vivo* or *in vitro* to thermal injury. The procedure was the same as above, that is intratesticular injection of boiling saline solution. The animals were serially studied between 1 – 4 weeks. The following was found: (1) With exception of positive results obtained with the sperm immobilization test, anaphylactic, precipitating and, fixing complement antisperm antibodies were absent. (2) Delayed hypersensitivity as revealed by skin test and inhibition of macrophage migration was positive from the second week simultaneously with testicular and epididymal damage resembling classical allergic orchitis. (3) Only homogenates from acutely thermally damaged testis, but not those from chronic sclerotic orchitis, provoked such a response. (4) Homogenates obtained from normal adult testis or from acute thermal nephritis gave negative results (MANCINI *et al.,* 1972) (Table 6).

These observations indicate that allergic orchitis may result in homologous guinea pigs without the addition of complete Freund's adjuvant. It has long been accepted that adjuvant mixed with normal testicular homogenate are both essential to obtain such a response. However, in our experiments, a single subcutaneous administration of the antigen provoked testicular alteration, delayed hypersensitivity and immobilization of sperm, without detectable circulating antisperm antibodies. Since the dermal inflammatory granuloma developing at sites of cutaneous sensitization has features analo-

Table 6. Immunologic response and testicular lesions developed in guinea pigs after homologous sensitization with normal or abnormal testicular homogenate without added adjuvants. [MANCINI, MAZZOLLI, and THIERER; Proc. Soc. exp. Biol. Med. 139, 991 (1972)].

Lot number	Animal sensitized with homogenate from	No. of animals	Days after sensiti-zation	Delayed skin test (mm)			Inhibition of macrophage migration (%)			Circulating antibodies		
				No. of positive	Mean	Range	No. of positive	Mean	Range	PCA-C. fix. precipit. No. of Positive	Immobil. test No. of positive	Testicular lesion No. of positive
1	3 days thermal orchitis	8	15	6/6	9.17	(7.5–11)	5/6	64	(51–77)	0/8	5/8	5/8
		9	30	9/9	8.5	(5.5–11)	6/6	64.5	(59–70)	0/9	0/9	7/9
2	1 month thermal orchitis	5	15	0/5	2	(1.5–3)	0/4	11	(5–18)	0/5	0/5	0/5
		6	30	0/6	1.7	(0.5–3)	0/4	8.7	(2–17)	0/6	0/6	0/6
3	Testis infiltrated *in vitro* with boiling saline	10	15	2/8	10.5	(10–11)	2/6	59.5	(56–63)	0/10	5/8	5/10
		8	30	6/8	9.3	(7–11)	5/5	67	(59–77)	0/8	0/6	5/8
4	Testis heated *in vitro* with boiling saline	6	15	0/6	2	(0.5–3.5)	0/6	6	(1–12)	0/6	2/6	3/6
		7	30	0/7	1.7	(0.5–3.5)	0/7	9.1	(5–17)	0/7	0/7	3/7
5	3 days thermal nephritis	5	15	0/5	1.8	(0.5–2)	0/4	8.5	(5–12)	0/5	0/5	0/5
		5	30	0/5	1.7	(0.5–2.5)	0/4	10.2	(4–18)	0/5	0/5	0/5
6	Normal testis	10	30	0/10	1.8	(0.5–3)	0/10	7.3	(3–17)	0/10	0/10	0/10

gous to those that have occurred after administration of complete Freund's adjuvant, the question arises as to whether or not the heat-denatured testicular homogenate used as antigenic stimulant and the resultant dermal granuloma are exclusively responsible for the immunologic and testicular damage. Specificity is supported by the absence of such immune response, following injections with testis not exposed to acute heat damage, but carrying only a chronic sclerotic area, normal testicular tissue, or kidney with thermal nephritis. As delayed hypersensitivity appears to be correlated with damage of seminiferous epithelium and with the remarkable intertubular mononuclear infiltration, attention is called to the predominant delayed reaction obtained in the absence of added adjuvant. More research is needed to clarify the nature of the testicular antigen induced by heat treatment and capable of provoking testicular injury in homologous animals and a consistent cell-mediated antibody response in absence of any adjuvant.

Autologous Sensitization with Thermal Orchitis Homogenate. Because in homologous experiments the transplantation antigens may have enhanced the antigenic potency of testis homogenate, attempts have been made to reproduce in an autologous model similar testicular lesions and immunologic responses. Adult noninbred guinea pigs were intradermally inoculated with their own testicular tissue, obtained by hemicastration and previously exposed *in vitro* to boiling saline. Inoculation with this material was made in a single dose in one site or by daily injection for 30 days, either in the same site or in different sites of the back; no Freund's adjuvant was used.

The following was observed: (1) sperm immobilizing and fixing complement tests were positive throughout in animals daily sensitized in the same site; in the remaining experiments results were erratic; (2) delayed hypersensitivity, as revealed by skin test and migration of macrophages, was positive in animals sensitized in the same site, whereas guinea pigs sensitized in different sites for an equal period of time exhibited similar but variable results; (3) in most of the animals daily sensitized in one site, the remaining testis developed typical lesions of allergic orchitis and inflammatory reaction in the epididymis parallel with humoral and cellular immunity responses (MAZZOLLI *et al.*, 1976).

The results demonstrate the high antigenic autologous potency, without added adjuvant, of an homogenate prepared from thermally injured testes, when sensitization is repeatedly performed in the same dermal site. This is supported by the fact that daily injections in the same site with an homogenate from thermally uninjured gonad do not elicit either testicular or immunologic response, but is at variance with the positive results obtained using normal gonadal tissue without adjuvants and inoculated during several months. In the latter experiment, the large number of injections needed may account for the "adjuvant function" of products derived from the irritated dermal tissue (BISHOP, 1961). The *in vivo* injured autologous testis daily inoculated in the same cutaneous site appears to be significantly correlated to a more complete and uniform response than homogenate made from *in vitro* thermally injured testis. Probably substances formed in the inflammatory reaction and present in the orchitis homogenate potentiate the antigenicity of a heat-injured tissue.

Daily doses injected in the same site seem to be essential; this differs from the homologous experiment, where only a single dose of the antigen was needed. It also points to the significance of the transplantation antigens in the homologous experiment; in this condition animals showed a granuloma at the site of skin sensitization. A similar dermal reaction was detected in the autologous condition where injections were daily performed in the same place; therefore the role of skin macrophages and mononuclear cells as primer structures in the chain of events in this autoimmune orchitis requires further study. Future investigations should also attempt to elucidate whether the antigenic potency of the heat-injured testis depends on altered antigens or whether some new antigens are formed.

Effect of Unilateral Traumatic Orchitis on the Contralateral Gonad. Thermal injury in one testis of adult guinea pigs is accompanied by lesions in the remaining gonad and antisperm antibodies. An attempt was therefore made to discover if other types of injury such as trauma, without added adjuvants, may produce similar results. Previous studies have described the reaction of the remnant tissue after partial removal of the testis. The resulting reaction is of a similar nature to that seen in allergic orchitis, judging by damage to seminiferous tubules, accumulation of mononuclear cells, binding of globulins to germinal cells, and PCA humoral antibodies (RAITSINA and NILOVSKY, 1967). Adult guinea pigs were submitted under general anesthesia to mechanical pressure on one of the testes; intensity of trauma was considered optimal when the gland lost its characteristic consistency. The animals were killed at 10 – 15, 30 – 48 and 55 – 90 days after injury. Histological study of the injured gonad as well as of the contralateral gland was made. Macrophage inhibition tests and serologic techniques were also performed. In the injured gonad there was destruction of a great part of tubules and inflammatory reaction mainly associated with polymorphonuclear leukocytes, hemorrhage, and necrosis during the first 2 weeks. This was followed by a diffuse accumulation of macrophages, mononuclear round cells, and juvenile fibroblasts in the subsequent period; in some cases this hyperplastic tissue exhibited features of an extensive granulomatous reaction. After two months, a fibrotic process began to replace most of the seminiferous tubules. In the contralateral gonad there were several focal lesions of germinal cells, sloughing, and cytolysis, together with interstitial accumulation of mononuclear round cells, at the time or after the appearance of granuloma in the injured testis. Thereafter there were no obvious changes in this gland. Delayed hypersensitivity was positive during that period, while humoral antibodies were detectable in very low titers (FAINBOIM et al., 1976).

It may be inferred from these observations that an inflammatory reaction as a result of traumatic injury induced in one testis may be paralleled, without addition of adjuvants, by previously described lesions in the other gland. The close chronologic correlation between testis lesions in the contralateral gland and a granulomatous reaction of the injured gonad points to the participation of macrophages and mononuclear cells in the processing and transference of antigens liberated at the site of germinal cell destruction. This interpretation is strengthened by the concomitant and predominant occurrence of positive delayed hypersensitivity. Similar cell accumulation in thermal orchitis and the positive results obtained in the passive intratesticular transference of

lymphocytes and macrophages from animals sensitized with testis plus adjuvants further reinforce this view (KANTOR and DIXON, 1972). Still more evidence is needed before one could categorically state that an immunologic mechanism has been set in mo-
tion and acts as mediator in this autologous traumatic spermatogenic damage.

8. Prevention of Immunologic Orchitis

It is well known that inhibition of the immune response can be obtained in various experimental systems by the use of cytostatic drugs, thymectomy, antilymphocyte serum, reduction of reactivity, or interference with the target organ and possible neutralization of histocompatibility antigens. The available information on allergic orchitis is summarized below.

Assuming that the potential damage involved in an autoimmune condition is initiated by the breakdown of natural tolerance against autoantigens, prevention could be attempted in several ways: (1) by induction of tolerance to the corresponding antigen, thus neutralizing or inhibiting the particular clone; (2) by passive transference of homologous antiserum; (3) by removing the thymus; (4) by administration of antimetabolites, cytostatic drugs, or corticosteroid hormones to block the reactivity of the immune cellular system; (5) by treatment with antilymphocyte serum to inhibit the response of mononuclear cells.

a) Tolerance

Some efforts have been made to induce tolerance toward testicular antigen, so that allergic orchitis is subsequently prevented by antigenic exposure, before immunologic competence develops in the neonate or the adult.

Neonatal Sensitization. Neonatal guinea pigs injected with homologous testicular homogenate from adult animals plus Freund's complete adjuvant exhibit aspermatogenesis after reaching maturity. Sensitization thus occurs early and there is an early release of humoral antibody detectable by PCA reaction. The processes of germinal epithelium differentiation and completion of spermatogenesis are not inhibited or prevented but germinal cell destruction follows later. Both testes tend to respond alike and unilateral castration during neonatal or adolescent stages has no effect on the aspermatogenic response of the remaining testis. It is clear that neonatal guinea pigs are immunologically competent as judged by their capacity to produce humoral antibody during the first week after birth. The extent of this capacity before birth and the degree to which it is developed shortly after, compared with that of the adult, can only be surmised. Immune tolerance in guinea pigs must thus be induced *in utero*. It therefore seems that this immunologic ability of neonatal animals may account for the initial phases of the aspermatogenic syndrome. It is unnecessary to postulate the persistence of the antigen for long periods, even though this might have been facilitated by the use of adjuvant and the injection into intracutaneous sites. This experiment supports the recognition hypothesis of forbidden clones above mentioned and suggests that different types of immunologic competence develop in sequence in young animals (BISHOP *et al.*, 1961).

Postnatal Sensitization. In some model systems it has been shown that the injection of large amounts of the respective antigen inhibits the immunological reactivity and induces tolerance in previously sensitized adult animals (MITCHISON, 1964). Following this concept, the possibility of induction of immunologic tolerance to organ-specific testicular antigen in previously immunized guinea pigs has been demonstrated. Results obtained indicate that immunologic tolerance can be induced by high doses of testicular antigen in guinea pigs, which had been subjected to immunization with testicular antigen added with complete Freund's adjuvant (CHUTNÁ and RYCHLÍKOVÁ, 1964 a). These animals responded by positive skin test and the production of PCA and cytotoxic antibodies. Evaluation of the spermatogenic process in animals treated in this way showed that further development of autoimmune damage to the testes is markedly inhibited as a result of immunologic tolerance. Cytologic studies of lymph nodes and spleen indicate that rapid differentiation and disappearance of cell types involved in the immune response, such as hemocytoblast and cells of plasmocyte series, take place after injection of high doses of antigen. Since in experiments of this type the antigen has been inoculated into animals which had already responded by antibody formation, antibodies could have interfered with the injected antigen, especially when it was given in repeated small doses. Furthermore, as tolerance is elicited more rapidly by high rather than small doses of antigen, evaluation of experiments indicates a more rapid onset of tolerance after injection of the given amount of antigen divided into high doses. The rapid progress of spermatogenesis approaching that of non-immunized controls suggests that the course of the autoimmune process is effectively slowed down in about half the number of animals used. The presence of 7S PCA antibodies in the guinea pigs in which the delayed skin sensitivity disappeared and the fact that no 19S cytotoxic antibodies were formed suggest that antibody response can be suppressed more easily than PCA anaphylactic reaction. As regards the cytologic changes in the lymph nodes and spleen, examination after the second high dose of antigens showed that the damaging effect manifested itself by the presence of degenerating and disintegrating cells, some of which could still be identified in the spleen as plasma cells and as small lymphocytes in the lymph nodes (CHUTNÁ and RYCHLÍKOVÁ, 1964 a). Since in these experiments autoimmune damage to the testes at the time of injection of the first doses of testicular antigen could be found in only 40% of the animals, it appears that immunologic tolerance delayed the further development of allergic orchitis in guinea pigs, which had not yet developed the disease at the time of the first dose.

Based on the induction of immunologic tolerance, the possibility of preventing the development of this autoimmune experimental disease was next attempted. Adult guinea pigs were immunized with testicular antigen in saline which produced PCA antibodies and immediate skin reaction, but no delayed hypersensitivity, humoral antibodies or autoimmune disease in the testes. Repeated inoculations prior to sensitization with the same antigen in complete Freund's adjuvant also resulted in the prevention of allergic orchitis in all the experimental animals (CHUTNÁ and RYCHLÍKOVÁ, 1964 b). It appears that the antibodies detectable by the PCA reaction were related to the presence of the immediate type of reaction but not the damage of germinal cells, which suggests that these antibodies may be associated with the prevention of this disease. Since the higher the dose of testis, in saline, inoculated, the greater the effectiveness of the suppression of immunologic aspermatogenesis, it is probable that, as in other systems, the excess antigen becomes bound to the effectors of the immune response and a blocking effect operates. Temporary suppression of similar autoimmune experimental diseases, such as encephalomyelitis (WAKSMAN, 1959 b; SHAW et al., 1960) and thyroiditis (JANKOVIC and FLAX, 1963), led the authors to think that a mechanism related to immunologic tolerance or enhancement-like effect is involved.

b) Passive Transference of Homologous Serum

Although there is a lack of sufficient experimental proof, a suggestion has been made that the enhancement-like mechanism participates in this phenomenon (CHUTNÁ and RYCHLIKOVÁ, 1964 b). This interpretation is reinforced by the prevention of immunologic encephalomyelitis after passive transfer of homologous antibodies detectable by complement fixation, which were not correlated with the intensity of this disease (PATERSON and HARWIN, 1963). An extension of the present concept of immune reaction, rejection reaction enhancement or facilitation reaction and their biological significance in the immunologic homeostasis in normal and pathologic conditions is discussed fully in a recent review (VOISIN, 1971).

The immunosuppressive effect of multiple small doses of normal nonimmune serum (heterologous, homologous, and isologous) on allergic orchitis, more evident in mice than in guinea pigs, accompanied by inhibition of cytotoxic antibodies but not of PCA and hemagglutinating types is probably due to a nonspecific mechanism (POKORNÁ and VÓJTISKOVÁ, 1966).

c) Thymectomy

Yet another approach to prevent the development of allergic orchitis is by thymectomy. Inhibition of immunologic encephalomyelitis in rats by early thymectomy seems to justify attempts in this direction (ARNASON et al., 1962). In order to see whether thymectomy would prevent the induction of or cause an interference with further development of the already established disease in adult animals, adult male mice were immunized with isologous testicular homogenate administered with Freund's adjuvant and thymectomized at varying stages. It was found that thymectomy provided marked protection if carried out not only before immunization at 5 weeks of age, but also between the inoculating doses at 8 and even 3 weeks later. Absence of thymus obviously accelerates recovery, since 4 weeks postoperationally the damage was significantly less than in the unoperated controls (VÓJTISKOVÁ and POKORNÁ, 1964).

d) Antimetabolites

Attempts to inhibit immunologic orchitis by drug treatment were based on the finding that purine analogues interfere with the formation of humoral antibodies. This led to extensive screening of various antimetabolites in relation to their inhibitory effects on the cellular type of immune response (SCHWARTZ and DAMESHEK, 1959). The immunosuppressive action of these drugs was tested in different experimentally induced autoimmune conditions, and clinical data on their use in diseases of a suspected autoimmune nature have been reported (PAGE et al., 1964). Immunologic aspermatogenesis induced in male mice could be inhibited by means of a 3-week regime of daily injections of amethopterin. The curative effect was achieved not only when the drug had been administerd one week after immunization, but also when the autoimmune seminiferous tubule lesions were fully developed. The disease did not reappear even when tested as late as 4 weeks after discontinuation of therapy. The serum of treated animals contained no cytotoxic or PCA antibodies. The therapeutic success might be accounted for by the drug-induced immunologic tolerance to the respective autoantigen. Both in amethopterin untreated and treated mice, the spleen exhibited amyloidosis. Two types of changes also appeared in the thymus in which reticular cells surrounded with lymphocytes and numerous spherical homogenous bodies of various sizes with nuclear staining affinity were detected (VÓJTISKOVÁ et al., 1965).

There is insufficient information on the effect of immunosuppressive agents such as alkylating substances, corticosteroid hormones or antilymphocyte serum in the prevention or suppression of allergic orchitis. However, it must be remembered that in animals (JACKSON et al., 1961) as well as in humans (CHEVIAKOFF et al., 1971) alkylating and cytostatic drugs have a direct deleterious effect on spermatogenesis.

II. Clinical Immunologic Orchitis

1. Antigenicity of Human Testis

Studies on the immunogenic properties of human material from different segments of the genital tract have been few, as compared with those carried out with animal tissues. This is understandable considering the difficulty of obtaining fresh tissue from autopsies or sufficient amounts from biopsies.

As described earlier, experiments performed over 60 years ago have indicated that extracts made from human testis were highly antigenic in heterologous sensitization. The antibodies produced in this way were demonstrated by their immobilizing and agglutinating properties. Lately, a component rich in proteins and carbohydrates has been identified in extract from human testis obtained at autopsy (KATSH, 1960 c). Antigenic potency was verified by sensitization in guinea pigs and corresponding antibodies were shown by precipitating technique and immunoelectrophoresis. These antibodies also cross-reacted with guinea pig testis antigens.

The autoantigenicity of human testis was further tested by using the immunofluorescent technique and histological sections of human testis from subjects with different types of endocrine and nonendocrine pathology. It was subsequently postulated that the localization of gamma-globulins in certain structures of the seminiferous tubular wall might be indirect evidence of testicular autoimmunity in man (DONDERO and ISIDORI, 1972).

a) Induced Allergic Orchitis

The antigenicity of human testis was confirmed more recently and examined in autologous and homologous sensitization procedures. To investigate the possible auto- or homoantigenic potency of the human testis, an attempt was made to induce allergic orchitis in man (MANCINI et al., 1965). These experiments were designed to examine the immunologic role of the human testis and to substantiate the supposition that antisperm autoantibodies may cause male infertility. Material was collected from patients with prostatic carcinoma who had had no previous treatment and were going to be castrated for therapeutic purposes. Autologous and homologous type of sensitization was performed on the patients of Group I, shown in Table 7. In the first case a testis was removed from one of the patients and served as the source of antigens to be self-injected. In the second case the same testicular material was injected into another patient. The first antigen used, a testicular homogenate (TH), was aseptically prepared from 5 g of tissue mixed with 1.5 ml complete Freund's adjuvant (CA) and 9.75 ml of saline solution. The second antigen was extracted from testis by the ammonium sulphate precipi-

Table 7. Correlation among antigenic stimuli, immunologic response, and testicular lesion in sensitized and unsensitized groups of patients after 6 weeks of inoculation.

(*TH*): Testicular homogenate. (*ASP*): Ammonium sulphate precipitated fraction. (*MUC*): Mucoprotein substance (*GLY*): Glycoprotein preparation. (*CA*): Complete Freund's adjuvant. (*IA*): Incomplete Freund's adjuvant. (*PCA*): Passive cutaneous anaphylactic test; number of (+) indicates diameter in cm. of the blue spot (*CFT*): Complement fixation test titers. (*GDT*): double agar diffusion technique; (+) indicates the presence of 1 line. (*AGCT*): Antiglobulin consumption test. Number of (+) is the positive reaction as expressed by absence of agglutination of red cells (negative Coombs test) in 2 or more of the 5 tubes containing the dilution between 1/80 and 1/1280 of the antiglobulin antisera. (Skin Test): diameter of the papulae, (+) equivalent to 1 cm. (immob. Test): Dilution of serum after 1 hour of incubation. (Immunofl. Test): Positive reaction of acrosome of germinal cells in testis sections. (Testic. lesion): Pos. indicates the presence of several foci of typical allergic orchitis. [MANCINI *et al.*, J. Clin. Endocr. Metab. **25**, 859 (1965)]

Patient group	Patient	Age	Antigenic stimuli	Type of sensitization	PCA	CFT	GDT	AGCT	Skin test	Immob. effect	Immunfl. test	Testic. lesion
I. Completely sensitized	1	59	TH +CA	Autolog.	+++	1/64	+	+++	+	1/64	Pos.	Pos.
	2	62	TH +CA	Homol.	+++	1/32	+	++++	+	1/120	Pos.	Pos.
	3	61	TH +CA	Autolog.	++	1/32	+	++	±	1/16	Pos.	Pos.
	4	60	TH +CA	Homol.	+	1/16	+	+	Neg.	1/16	Neg.	Pos.
	5	62	ASP +CA	Homol.	+	1/16	Neg.	Neg.	Neg.	1/8	Neg.	Neg.
	6	63	ASP =CA	Homol.	±	Neg.	Neg.	+	+	Neg.	Neg.	Neg.
	7	59	ASP =CA	Homol.	++	1/64	+	++	+	1/64	Pos.	Pos.
	8	62	MUC =CA	Homol.	Neg.	Neg.	Neg.	Neg.	Neg.	Neg.	Neg.	Neg.
	9	64	MUC =CA	Homol.	Neg.	Neg.	Neg.	Neg.	Neg.	Neg.	Neg.	Neg.
	10	65	MUC =CA	Homol.	±	1/16	Neg.	+	±	Neg.	Neg.	Neg.
	11	58	GLY =CA	Homol.	Neg.	Neg.	Neg.	Neg.	Neg.	Neg.	Neg.	Neg.
	12	62	GLY =CA	Homol.	+	Neg.	Neg.	Neg.	+	1/32	Neg.	Neg.
	13	63	GLY =CA	Homol.	+	1/32	Neg.	+	+	1/16	Pos.	Neg.

Table 7 (continued)

Patient group	Patient	Age	Antigenic stimuli	Type of sensitization	Immunological tests					Immob. effect	Immunfl. test	Testic. lesion
					PCA	CFT	GDT	AGCT	Skin test			
II. Incompletely sensitized	14	58	CA alone		Neg.	Neg.	Neg.	Neg.	Neg.	1/8	Neg.	Neg.
	15	60	IA alone		+	Neg.	Neg.	Neg.	±	Neg.	Neg.	Neg.
	16	62	TH alone	Homol.	Neg.	Neg.	Neg.	Neg.	Neg.	Neg.	Neg.	Neg.
	17	62	TH +IA	Autolog.	±	Neg.	Neg.	Neg.	±	Neg.	Neg.	Neg.
	18	65	ASP +IA	Homol.	±	Neg.	Neg.	Neg.	±	1/8	Neg.	Neg.
	19	62	MUC +IA	Homol.	Neg.	Neg.	Neg.	Neg.	Neg.	Neg.	Neg.	Neg.
III. nonsensitized	20	64			Neg.	Neg.	Neg.	Neg.	Neg.	Neg.	Neg.	Neg.
	21	63			+	Neg.	Neg.	Neg.	Neg.	1/8	Neg.	Neg.
	22	59			Neg.	Neg.	Neg.	Neg.	Neg.	Neg.	Neg.	Neg.
	23	58			Neg.	Neg.	Neg.	Neg.	Neg.	Neg.	Neg.	Neg.
	24	60	None		±	Neg.	Neg.	Neg.	±	1/8	Neg.	Neg.
	25	61			+	Neg.	Neg.	Neg.	Neg.	Neg.	Neg.	Neg.
	26	62			+	Neg.	Neg.	Neg.	Neg.	Neg.	Neg.	Neg.
	27	60			Neg.	Neg.	Neg.	Neg.	±	Neg.	Neg.	Neg.
	28	61			Neg.	Neg.	Neg.	Neg.	Neg.	Neg.	Neg.	Neg.
	29	63			Neg.	Neg.	Neg.	Neg.	Neg.	Neg.	Neg.	Neg.

tation procedure (ASP) and lyophilized. Three different doses, 50, 100, and 300 mg, mixed with 1.5 ml of Freund's adjuvant, were injected into three different patients. The third antigen, a mucoprotein (MUC), isolated from testicular tissue was supplied by Dr. S. KATSH (Denver, USA). The fourth antigen, a glycoprotein substance (GLY), was also extracted from human testis (MANCINI, 1968 b). Three doses of 50, 80, and 100 mg mixed with the same adjuvant were injected into another three patients. An incomplete sensitization was performed on six patients of Group II; complete (CA) or incomplete Freund's adjuvant (IA) alone, in doses of 1.5 ml, and testicular antigens alone or mixed with incomplete adjuvant were administered to patients of this group. In all cases of Group I and II biopsies were taken from the reacted skin at the site of immunization, after 1, 2 and 3 months. Ten patients of Group III were not sensitized and served as control. In order to detect the presence of circulating antibodies against testicular antigens and seminal spermatozoa, the passive cutaneous anaphylactic (PCA), the double agar diffusion, the hemagglutination, the Steffen antiglobulin consumption and the sperm immobilization and complement fixing tests were applied (Table 7). As antigen, sonicated washed spermatozoa provided by normal donors, autologous and homologous testicular homogenate, ASP and MUC were used. Specificity was checked using normal serum, absorption of the immune serum with testicular and other tissue antigens extracted from liver and kidney. To detect a delayed type of sensitization, a skin test was performed every 20 days after immunization, using a sterilized suspension of the spermatozoal or testicular antigens. Biopsies from the reacted skin at 48 and 72 hours were used for microscopic studies. Testicular biopsies were obtained from patients of Groups I and II, at 20, 30, 40, and 50 days after sensitization, followed by final castration after 2 to 3 months. Testicular tissue was processed for routine microscopic and immunofluorescent studies. The direct and indirect immunofluorescent method was performed using the patient's normal and immune sera.

Results obtained indicated that auto- or homologous sensitization could be induced in human beings using testicular homogenate or other complex antigen such as ASP, and with less certainty with MUC or GLY plus complete Freund's adjuvant. This was substantiated by immunologic, histological, and histoimmunochemical findings in the sensitized subjects. The reactions were not detectable after sensitization in the group of partially sensitized patients, or in nonsensitized control patients. It therefore seems reasonable to assume that the germinal cell destruction detected in the testis is an induced allergic or immunologic reaction. The fact that only 6 out of 13 patients clearly responded to immunization, that antibodies were of low titer and testicular lesions of moderate severity may be explained by the minimal amount of antigens used. This was particularly applicable in cases sensitized with ASP, MUC and GLY, where a slight response has only been achieved with higher doses. It must be taken into account that the patients studied, due either to age or to carcinoma, may have had a less reactive immune system, or were more susceptible to autologous sensitization to TH, as was the case in 2 out of 4 patients. The histological findings in the sensitizing cutaneous granuloma, the low levels of circulating antibodies, the fixed cell type antibodies revealed by positive skin test (Figs. 28 – 29), and the testicular lesions, were analogous to those encountered in animals. All these facts suggest the induction of a delayed type of cellular immunity reaction. The circulating antibodies (precipitating, anti-globulin consumption, PCA and complement fixing types) have been induced transiently by the inoculated antigens. Skin test, and more conspicuously the PCA, were in our cases apparently less specific than the other techniques. This is borne out by the unexplained erratic appearance of positive reactions in the control groups of patients. Since in some cases the patient's own testicular tissue (TH) was used in the sensitization and homologous procedures, and TH, ASP, MUC, GLY, or seminal spermatozoa as antigens in

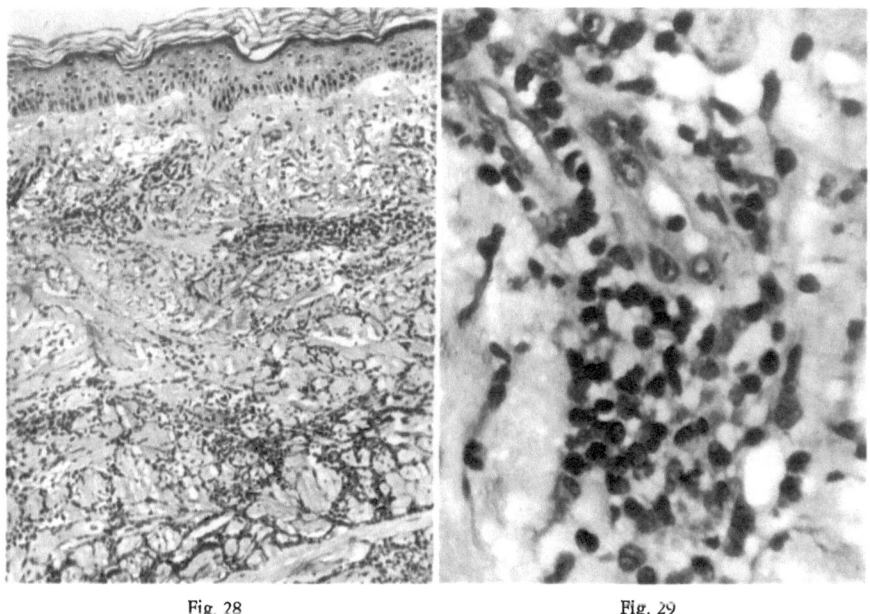

Fig. 28   Fig. 29

Fig. 28. Biopsy taken at site of skin test in sensitized patient 2 of Group I, after 72 hours of intradermal injection of free human homologous spermatozoa. Dermal reaction shows collagen edema, numerous fibroblast cells, and perivascular infiltration of mononuclear cells. H & E. ×110 [MANCINI, ALONSO, SARACENI, BACHMANN, LAVIERI and NEMIROVSKY; J. Clin. Endocr. Metab. 25, 859 (1965)]

Fig. 29. Same as in Fig. 28 at higher magnification. An arteriole with swollen wall and hypertrophied endothelium surrounded by accumulation of mononuclear cells and histiocytes. H & E. × 800 [MANCINI et al.; J. Clin. Endocr. Metab. 25, 859 (1965)]

the serological techniques and for the skin test, antisperm homo- and autoantibodies were elicited. Therefore, according to comparative results obtained with TH, ASP, MUC, and GLY it seemed that the two latter substances, since they are chemically better defined entities, should be more potent antigens; but this has not been the case in our experiments. Marked testicular lesions, present only in some patients of Group I, resembled those seen in sensitized animals. Congestion and serous edema accompanied by sloughing and cytolysis of germinal cells were the predominant inflammatory fea-

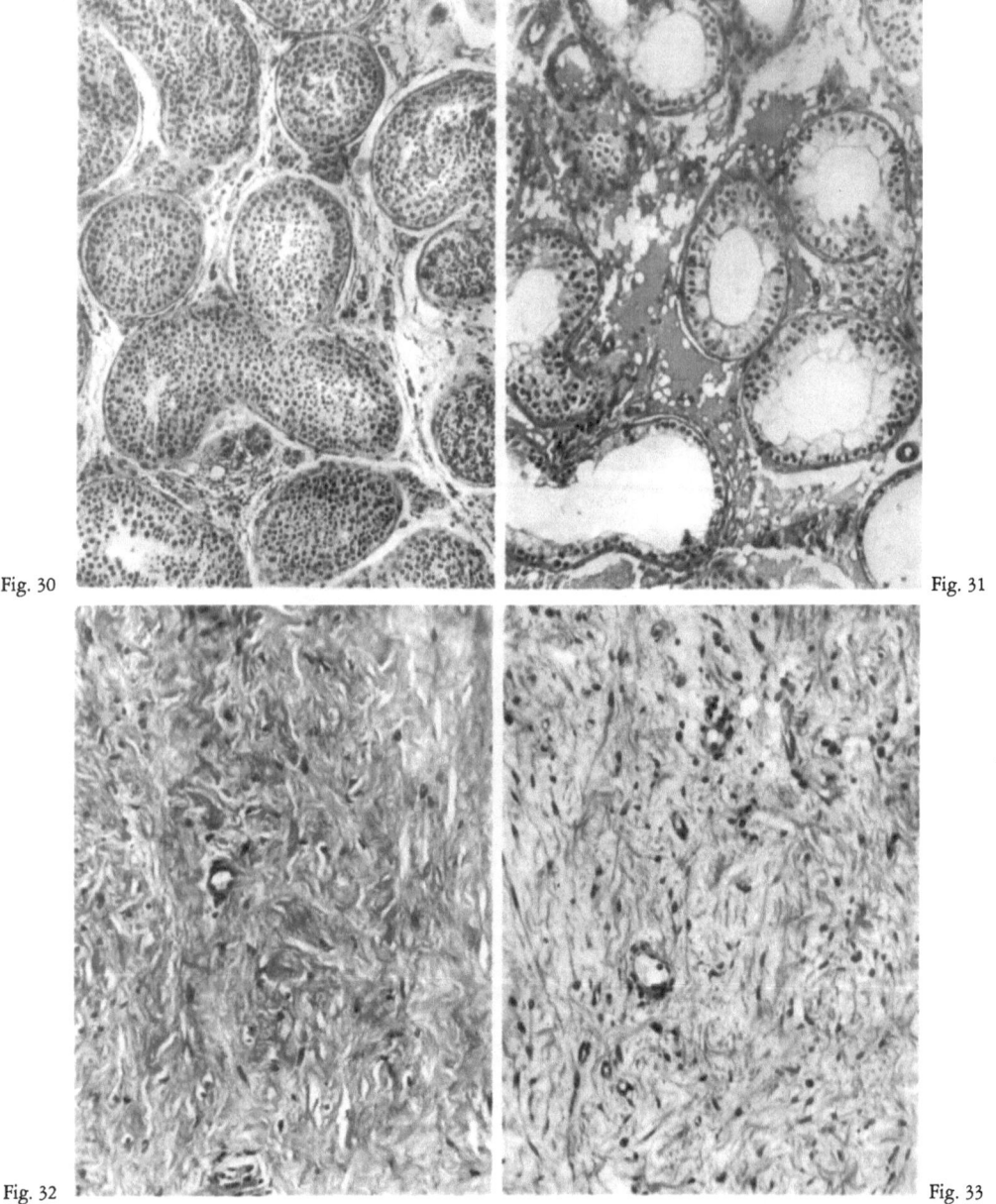

Fig. 30. Testis biopsy of patient 2 from Group I before sensitization. Nearly normal structures in seminiferous tubules content and intertubular spaces as well. H & E. × 120 [MANCINI et al.; J. Clin. Endocr. Metab. 25, 859 (1965)]

Fig. 31. Testis biopsy of same patient 40 days after sensitization. Seminiferous tubules show variable degrees of sloughing of germinal cells. Intertubular spaces appear somewhat wider and filled with an accumulation of plasmalike material. Clumps of Leydig cells and small vessels are normal. H & E. × 120 [MANCINI et al.; J. Clin. Endocr. Metab. 25, 859 (1965)]

Fig. 32. Tunica albuginea of testis of same patient before sensitization. Connective tissue with well packed collagen fibers and bundles, as well as normal cells and vessels. H & E. × 240 [MANCINI et al.; J. Clin. Endocr. Metab. 25, 859 (1965)]

Fig. 33. Inner zone of tunica albuginea of same patient 40 days after sensitization. Interfibrillar collagen edema, dissociated collagen fibers, and diffuse infiltration of mononuclear round cells. H & E. × 240 [MANCINI et al.; J. Clin. Endocr. Metab. 25, 859 (1965)]

tures (Figs. 30 – 33). Nonspecific lesions, such as arrest of spermatogenesis and fibrosis, which are commonly seen in subjects at this age, were observed either before or after sensitization in the remaining patients of Groups I, II, and III. The substantially different picture reinforces the significance of the inflammatory response found in biopsies after sensitization, as far as vascular phenomena and lysis of germinal cells are concerned. The mild character of this transient allergic orchitis is also confirmed by the absence of gross clinical signs in the gonad. The localization of fluorescent immunoglobulins in the perinuclear area of spermatids and acrosome of spermatozoa of the patient's own testis (Figs. 34 – 35) also suggests the presence of an anti-acrosomic globulin factor (MANCINI *et al.,* 1965; MANCINI, 1968 b).

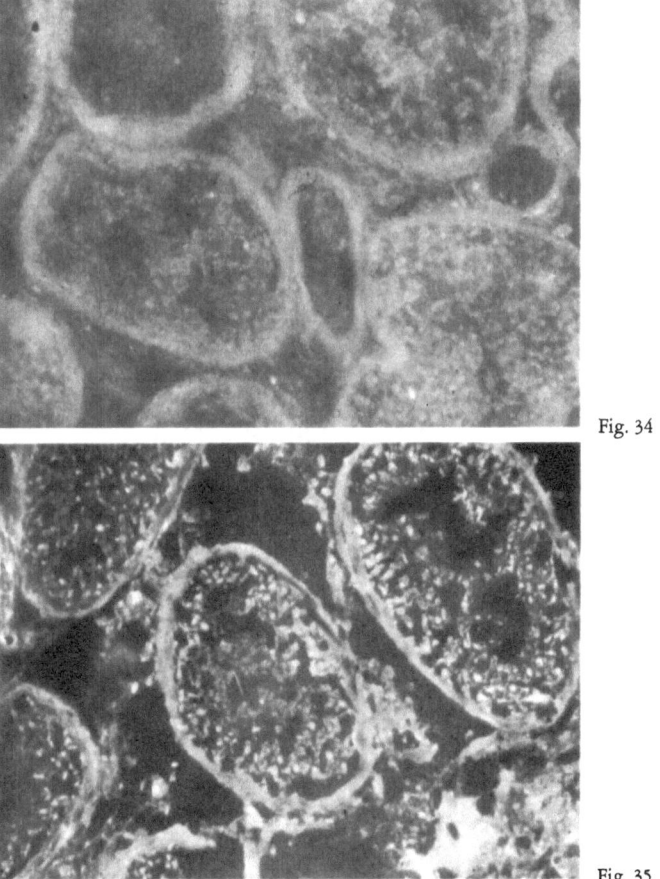

Fig. 34

Fig. 35

Fig. 34. Section of testis biopsy of same patient incubated with homologous normal serum followed by labeled serum against human gamma globulin. No positive fluorescence is seen in the seminiferous tubules or in intertubular spaces. Immunofluorescent technique. × 220 [MANCINI *et al.*; J. Clin. Endocr. Metab. 25, 859 (1965)]

Fig. 35. Same testis biopsy as in Fig. 34. Section incubated with patient's own serum followed by labeled rabbit serum against human gamma-globulin. Positive reaction in germinal cells, spermatids, and spermatozoa. Some moderate or weak staining also seen in peritubular structures and vessel walls. × 220 [MANCINI *et al.*; J. Clin. Endocr. Metab. 25, 859 (1965)]

2. Antigenicity of Human Spermatozoa

Human spermatozoa, like other animal sperm cells, contain several different antigens, but in most studies for antibodies against these cells this complex situation has largely been ignored. For instance, whole human semen or seminal spermatozoa have proved to be antigenic in sensitized animals. Species-specific antibodies have been demonstrated by complement fixation and immobilizing tests, and even different types of sperm agglutination have been observed (MUDD and MUDD, 1929; HENLE et al., 1938).

Human semen or sperm cells have also been claimed to be a highly potent antigen in homologous sensitization. One of the first attempts to obtain humoral antisperm antibodies in humans, and subsequently to achieve infertility has been performed in adult women who had been inoculated with sperm from normal fertile donors (BASKIN, 1932).

Lately, there has been a renewal of interest in this topic based on the assumption that female or male infertility could be correlated with the existence of antisperm antibodies. As these antibodies show a number of properties detectable by different procedures, immunobiologic methods for detecting antisperm factors similar to those described in animal experiments will be reviewed.

a) Immobilization Test

The sperm immobilization test due to its simplicity and specificity seems to be a reliable one and is performed as follows. Fresh normal semen (60×10^6 sperm per ml.) which contains more than 80% motile spermatozoa, is used; 0.25 ml of twofold serial dilution of inactivated tested human serum is added to 0.025 ml of fresh normal semen and 0.05 ml of fresh complement (guinea pig serum). The incubation lasts 60 min. at $32°$ C after which the percentage of immotile spermatozoa is counted. One control experiment running at the same time is done using normal human serum, and another control experiment without complement. When motile spermatozoa are less than 10% of the control preparation, the result is considered positive.

Specificity of the immobilizing factor in serum was checked by absorption procedure using (1) human semen, (2) human aspermic ejaculate and human kidney, (3) heat elution of sperm immobilizing factor from incubated spermatozoa with patient's serum, (4) iodination with I^{131} of patient's serum and normal globulin obtained by salting out procedure, (5) *in vitro* purification and *in vitro* adsorption of binding substance in patient's serum. In this case gamma-globulin from a patient's serum was labeled with I^{131} and then incubated with spermatozoa. After incubation the mixture was centrifuged and washed. The spermatozoa were again incubated in heated saline solution and the percentage of dissociation of labeled material was calculated. The dissociation supernatant was incubated with freshly washed spermatozoa and sedimented. Lastly, from the count of total supernatant and the sedimented sperm, percentage adsorption of the purified factor on spermatozoa was calculated.

These findings indicate that the immobilizing factor displays antibody-like behavior. It is specifically absorbed with spermatozoa but not with aspermic seminal fluid or kidney. It behaves like a high molecular substance and fractionates in the gammaglobulin portion. Once attached to spermatozoa it can be eluted by heating and needs complement to immobilize sperm. When I^{131} labeled patient's gamma-globulin was purified by elution from spermatozoa, it localized on spermatozoa more than twice as much as labeled globulin from normal serum (ISOJIMA et al., 1968).

b) Agglutination Test

Agglutination of spermatozoa in some cases of male unexplained sterility has drawn the attention of various authors (KIBRICK et al., 1952; WILSON, 1954). Recognition of two classes of agglutination was soon accepted, one spontaneous with no clearly defined etiology, and the other induced by human serum or seminal plasma, more significant for its pathogenicity (WILSON, 1954). Microscopic and macroscopic techniques have been worked out to visualize this phenomenon and the patient's serum or seminal plasma and spermatozoa were used. Microscopically two types of sperm agglutination were observed, namely head-to-head and tail-to-tail, but sometimes also a tail-to-head type.

Various alternative procedures for animal and human spermatozoa have been proposed (KIBRICK et al., 1952; FRANKLIN and DUKES, 1964). A routine procedure is as follows. Fresh unwashed spermatozoa from ejaculates are used which retain their motility. The sperm cell suspension is adjusted to 10×10^6/ml with Baker's buffer. It is mixed at $37°$ C with an equal volume of 10% gelatin to provide the test antigen. An equal volume of the patient's serum tested or normal serum is added. The samples are gently mixed and transferred with a Pasteur pipette to a small tube 3.0 mm in diameter, avoiding the trapping of air bubbles. The tubes are incubated for 1 hr at $37°$ C. To obtain clear differentiation they must be observed after 2 hours. An alternative method, called the capillary tube technique, was also proposed. In this case, the incubations are made in glass capillaries, 1 – 2 mm in diameter. Equal volumes of the sperm suspension and a suitable dilution of the serum tested are mixed in a small tube; this mixture is aspirated into the capillary. Concentration of spermatozoa may range between 40×10^6/ml to 80×10^6/ml and the mixture is incubated at $22-25°$ C. Each capillary is quickly sealed at the lower end with a small amount of soft putty. Best results are obtained with spermatozoa that has been washed and resuspended in either saline or Baker's buffer. As a result of the washing the sperm are immotile, but experiments using both types of spermatozoa show that results are independent of motility (SHULMAN and HEKMAN, 1971).

One of the difficulties encountered with the agglutination method is the nonspecific type of agglutination and the fact that agglutination may not be the result of antibody activity (BOETTCHER and KAY, 1969). These points have recently been reviewed (SHULMAN and HEKMAN, 1971) and several factors involved in the agglutination reaction discussed. It is striking that a much better agglutinating activity is obtained by using well-washed spermatozoa. This is presumably due to the removal of a large quantity of seminal plasma antigens capable of interfering with the sperm reaction. The advantage of using room temperature for incubation and the low number of spermatozoa needed are among parameters which probably deserve further study. Regarding the antibody nature of the agglutinating activity of a given serum, it has long been established that this factor is heat resistant, absorbable by packed spermatozoa, detectable in the gamma-globulin fraction after preparative paper electrophoresis and removable by absorption with semen. The serum does not agglutinate erythrocytes, leukocytes, or thrombocytes. ABO and Rh blood group differences between sera and spermatozoa do not influence the agglutinating effect (RÜMKE and HELLINGA, 1959). No precipitating antibodies have been observed in cases of sperm agglutinating sera using seminal plasma as antigen and no gamma-globulin fixation on spermatozoa (BANDHAUER, 1966; CRUICKSHANK and STUART-SMITH, 1959).

Male sera showing sperm agglutination have been studied (FJALLBRANDT, 1968 a) by absorption with seminal spermatozoa, with A and B blood group substances, by filtration on Sephadex G-200 and by reduction with mercaptoethanol and incubation at 56° C for 30 min. In addition, the agglutinating property was determined in the presence of complement, as well as by the levels of IgG, IgA, and IgM in the sera of patients and of normal men. Absorption with normal spermatozoa isolated from ejaculates completely exhausted the agglutinating activity, but it only removed the immobilizing activity present in the same serum. Absorption with blood group isoantigens did not modify the antibody reaction (FJALLBRANDT, 1968 a). Furthermore, the specificity of sperm agglutinins as far as sperm or seminal plasma are concerned has been checked (DUCKES and FRANKLIN, 1958). The sera of three patients with strong sperm agglutinating titers were selected. Serial twofold dilutions were prepared and each dilution was then absorbed with freeze-dried pooled seminal plasma. This procedure did not reduce significantly the agglutinating titer, whereas adsorption with sperm cells from spermatocele had a pronounced effect on the agglutinating activity. This experiment seems to indicate that only spermatozoal own antigens, and not the coating ones, are able to interfere with agglutinin antibodies.

The agglutinating property is mainly of the 7S type. A weak agglutination has been found in the first peak of certain sera and there may therefore be some agglutinating activity in molecules of a larger size. The results of mercaptoethanol reduction suggest that these antibodies represent only a minor part of the activity of the serum proteins. There is no change in activity after mercaptoethanol treatment and it may be concluded that 19S antibodies are not associated with sperm agglutination. The presence of complement does not influence the reaction at all. In the sera which revealed significant titers of agglutination, levels of IgG and IgM were significantly higher than in sera with no demonstrable activity (FJALLBRANDT, 1968 b).

c) Cytotoxicity Test

The cytotoxicity test has been proposed as a reliable technique for the detection of antisperm antibodies in humans. As in the case of the technique used in research, it is based on a test which had been worked out previously for leukocyte antibodies. The index of cytotoxicity is assessed by the uptake of Trypan blue by damaged spermatozoa in the presence of specific antiserum and complement. As substrate, only donor semen samples which have been freshly obtained, with a sperm count of around 10^8/ml and very good motility, must be used. The normal serum as control and the experimental serum to be tested should be heated at 56° C to destroy complement activity. Fresh human AB serum is used as a source of complement. One drop each of sperm suspension and serum, and two drops of complement, are mixed in a test tube and incubated at 37° C. Two more drops of complement are then added. After 90 min. of incubation one drop of Trypan blue is added. Centrifugation follows and from the sediment slide smears are prepared. The spermatozoa which have survived the incubation with the test serum appear unstained as luminous bodies; spermatozoa which have been killed during incubation are colored blue. Since cytotoxic antibodies are complement dependent, the test should be repeated with the positive sera in the absence of complement, to prove that the spermatotoxic activity of these sera was due to antibodies and not to any other cytotoxic complement independent substance.

Studies on the localization of the sperm cytotoxic activity in different immunoglobulin fractions are not available. It has been postulated that only cytotoxic antibodies to sperm can affect spermatogenesis or the motility of the spermatozoa; therefore the findings of a strong spermatotoxic activity in the sera of certain infertile patients, showing head-to-head type of agglutination, reinforce this hypothesis (HAMERLYNCK and RÜMKE, 1968).

d) Nature of Antigens

Apart from immunobiologic techniques, the serologic methods have provided an interesting source of information and identification of sperm antigens. Using the double gel precipitation test and rabbit antibodies against washed human spermatozoa, seven different antigens were described, four of which were also present in seminal plasma (RAO and SADRI, 1959). Later, the presence of antigens common to spermatozoa and seminal plasma as well as testicular tissue was confirmed (OTANI et al., 1965).

Coating Antigens. One of the antigens common to seminal plasma and spermatozoa seems to be lactoferrin, a substance secreted by seminal vesicles and probably one of the most potent antigens of human sperm. The presence of this antigen on the surface of spermatozoa was confirmed by agglutination and immobilization experiments and fluorescent antibody tests, using antiseminal plasma, antilactoferrin, and antimilk antibodies. For these tests the sperm cells were freed from seminal plasma by applying the capillary method referred to above. All these antisera agglutinated and immobilized the spermatozoa. This effect could be blocked by previous absorption of antisera with seminal plasma and washed sperm. Lactoferrin only inhibits the effect of antimilk serum and partially that of antiseminal plasma; this suggests the existence of other coating antigens in this material. Immunofluorescence shows staining of the head of sperm cells with both antimilk and antilactoferrin, but although absorption with seminal plasma diminishes the reaction, lactoferrin fails to do so (HEKMAN and RÜMKE, 1969).

The possibility that a great part of the antigenic material of spermatozoa is taken up during sperm transit is supported by the following findings. (1) Antisera against ejaculated spermatozoa, while showing strong, positive reactions with ejaculated spermatozoa, were completely negative when tested with epididymal sperm. In addition, antisera against seminal plasma also gave strong positive reactions with ejaculated spermatozoa but were totally negative with epididymal spermatozoa (WEIL and RODENBURG, 1962). (2) Sperm cells extracted from spermatocele lack the antigenicity which characterizes the seminal spermatozoa. This was proved by direct and cross-reactions performed with heterologous antihuman semen, antisperm or seminal plasma antibodies in double agar gel diffusion and complement fixation techniques (WEIL et al., 1956).

These findings formed the basis of the concept that one or several seminal plasma proteins of differing nature interact and are attached to the surface membranes of the spermatozoa, constituting the so-called coating antigens. This coating provides the cells with antigenic properties which dominate the immunologic behavior of seminal spermatozoa, properties that are not apparently present in the immature spermatozoa in the testis. The protein film is firmly attached to the spermatozoa and only traces can be released by various physical and chemical methods. Using rabbit antiserum against human seminal plasma or washed seminal spermatozoa, the coating antigens are detectable in higher dilution by complement fixation. They are quite stable in seminal plasma kept at 40° C or below 0° C; coating antigens are nondialyzable, resistant to heat up to 80° C and insoluble in the common organic solvent (WEIL, 1965). Further details about the chemical nature of coating antigens will be given in the next chapter.

Soluble and Insoluble Antigens. To examine how firmly the so-called coating antigens are attached to the spermatozoa, a gradual extraction procedure was applied based on washing with saline, followed by repeated washings with distilled water. With this method it is possible to extract water-soluble and insoluble antigenic components, independently of their physicochemical binding to the surface or deeper membranes of spermatozoa. After twenty successive washings with distilled water the extracted product was called "soluble fraction", the remaining material being considered as "relatively insoluble". Various by-products were obtained by successive precipitations and centrifugations at different speeds; chemical analyses were performed and control of diffusible proteins was performed by disc electrophoresis. The soluble fraction had a high concentration of proteins, lipids and carbohydrates, whereas the insoluble one showed the presence of nucleoproteins and a low concentration of proteins and carbohydrates.

Cross-reactions, using the agar diffusion test were noted between the insoluble fraction, the soluble one, and seminal plasma, against anti-seminal plasma and anti-insoluble fraction antibodies, suggesting the existence of common antigenic groups. Immuno-electrophoresis showed three arcs when the insoluble fraction reacted with anti-insoluble and anti-seminal plasma sera (SCACCIATI and MANCINI, 1975).

The fact that water can extract proteins and carbohydrates after repeated washings indicates that this material passes through the external membrane of the sperm cell and that water is necessary to enable this transport. The release of nondialysable substances after washing and freezing and the loss of proteins from ram spermatozoa have been demonstrated before (QUINN et al., 1969). It is conceivable that extractable material is bound to the membranes by some nonchemical linkage. The insoluble fraction indicated by disc electrophoresis that many of its proteins are highly diffusible. The interesting finding by the immunodiffusion test of two lines which do not react with anti-seminal plasma serum and which are more readily extractable than those common to seminal plasma and the soluble fraction, suggests the presence of "intrinsic" antigens. Another explanation may be the existence of different partition coefficients for these antigens, the spermatozoa, and the solvent employed (SCACCIATI and MANCINI, 1975). Solubilization of human spermatozoa using trypsin and/or dithioerythrol results in the decondensation and swelling of sperm heads. Thereby, an antigen, a protamine formed by 47 amino acids with a molecular weight of 6000 was isolated. This new antigen is able to fix IgG antibodies from sperm-agglutinating sera. This antigen does not appear to be related to any other present in the sperm head (KOLK et al., 1974; PATEL and SHULMAN, 1974). There is evidence that human spermatozoa do not need to be coated and capacitated in order to achieve fertilization. It has been claimed that successful pregnancies have followed artificial insemination with "uncoated" spermatozoa obtained from the urine of men, in whom there was an anatomic condition causing the voiding of spermatozoa into the bladder, or from the spermatocele (PIKO, 1967).

e) Immunohistochemical Localization of Antigens

Evidence concerning the existence of antigens in human spermatozoa has been mainly demonstrated by the induction of different antibodies endowed with biological properties and immunoserologic tests, whereas the localization of antigens in the structures of these cells was verified by immunohistochemical methods.

An early attempt was made (FELTKAMP et al., 1965) using sera of patients with sperm-agglutinating activity to which was added rabbit antihuman globulin conjugated with fluorescein isothiocyanate; smears of semen from normal donors diluted in phosphate buffer and centrifuged were used as substrate. The same procedure was applied to tissue sections of human testis obtained at autopsy soon after death. To investigate the deposition of the complement, the technical conditions were the same, except for the previous inactivation of the serum to be tested, and the addition of a fresh human serum blood group AB as a source of complement. Various types of fluorescent stain-

ing were seen in the area of the acrosome, in the whole head, the posterior part of
the head, the midpiece, and the main-piece or combination. On testicular sections only
the head and tail staining were distinguishable; sometimes, the entire sperm cell showed bright fluorescence. It is clear that there is a positive correlation between agglutination and fluorescent staining. In nearly all instances the mature sperm was stained
but a clear correlation between the agglutination type and the localization of fluorescence has not been found. The reactivity of sperm in the testis sections suggests that an
antigen of testicular origin exists similar to that present in the ejaculate. It is thus un-
likely that fluorescent antibodies (gamma-globulin) are directed against the coating antigens. Specificity was substantiated by negative results with normal or conjugated anti-
B2A and anti-B2M sera. The various patterns of fluorescence observed probably mean
that different antigens related to each other are present in spermatozoa.

Peroxidase Labeling. Almost simultaneously, two more reports have recently been
published which corroborate and amplify these findings. In the first (MANCINI *et al.,*
1971), a study of the development and localization of antigenic sites in human spermatozoa during transport through the genital tract was performed with the aid of a new
label for antibodies, namely the horseradish peroxidase (NAKANE and PIERCE, 1967).
Different sera were obtained as follows, by sensitization of adult rabbits with human
materials: antiseminal plasma, anti-washed seminal spermatozoa, antitesticular proteins
(ammonium sulphate precipitated fraction from germinal cells), antiserum proteins,
antiserum albumin, anti-immunoglobulins G, A and M, anti-beta-lipoprotein, and anti-
human testis collagen. All the control procedures usually performed in immunohistochemical techniques were included. Reactivity of these sera was checked by complement fixation and hemagglutination tests. Specificity of the histochemical techniques was controlled by absorption with corresponding antigens. Smears of spermatozoa
from ejaculates of normal donors, testis section from biopsies of fertile adult subjects,
and smears of spermatozoa from epididymis and spermatocele (obtained by puncture
during surgical interventions) were used. With antiseminal plasma, only spermatozoa
showed a positive reaction in the head cap or acrosome in seminiferous tubules of the
testis. The cells obtained from spermatocele and epididymis exhibited a more intense
reaction in the acrosome and occasionally in the postacrosomal area and neck. In seminal spermatozoa, a more intense staining in all areas described above was detectable, but
in no case was there a positive reaction observed in the tail. With anti-washed sperm
serum, only the acrosome appeared distinctly stained in the testis and in the epididymis, but in seminal spermatozoa both the acrosome and neck region reacted clearly.
With the antiprotein testicular fraction, a reaction was obtained in the acrosome and
neck of cells recovered from the testis and epididymis, which was less easily identifiable
in seminal smears. With antiserum proteins, staining was detected only in the acrosome
in sperm from ejaculates and it was very faint in preparations from testis and epididymis. A similar result was evident when antiserum against albumin or anti-beta-lipoprotein was used. With the exception of a slight positive reaction seen with anti-gam-
ma-globulin in seminal sperm, all the remaining sera gave negative results (Fig. 36).
All the reacted areas disappeared when the spermatozoa were washed in saline or distilled water for 30 min.

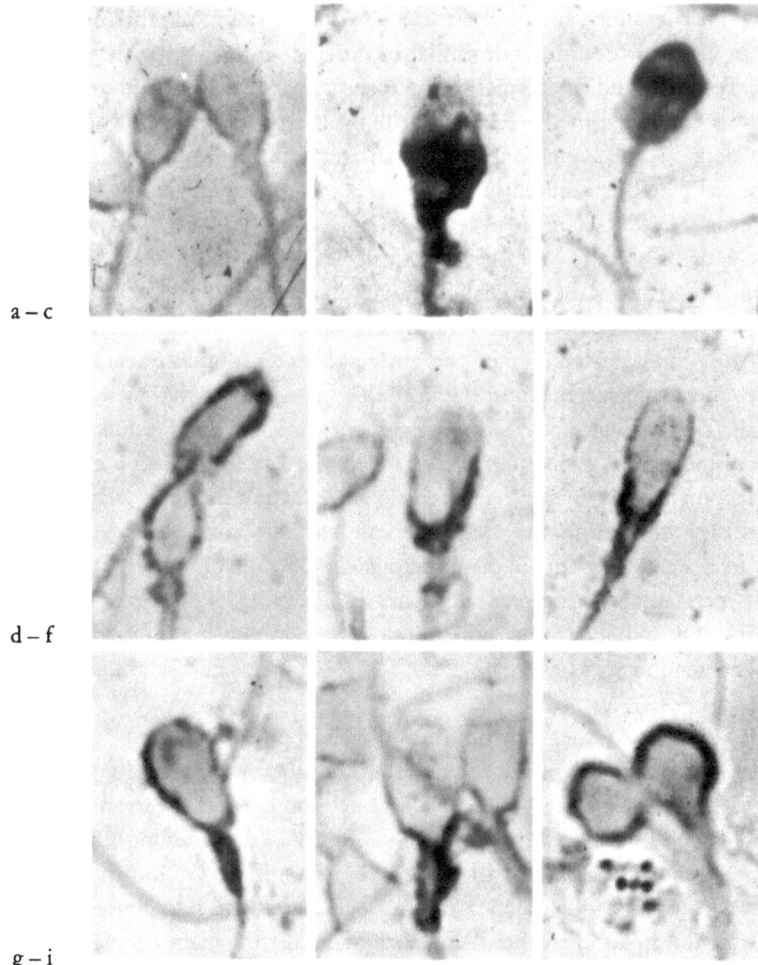

a – c

d – f

g – i

Fig. 36. Immunohistochemical reaction (black areas) between human spermatozoa and different antibodies labeled with peroxidase. × 1100. a): Control preparation incubated with rabbit anti-seminal plasma serum previously absorbed with sperm extract, followed by labeled goat globulin against rabbit gamma globulin. (b – h): Experimental preparation incubated with rabbit antiseminal plasma serum followed by labeled goat globulin against rabbit gamma globulin. (i): experimental preparation incubated with antihuman serum proteins followed by labeled goat globulin against human serum albumin. (a): no reaction detectable. (b): reaction in equatorial segment, post head cap and neck. (c): staining in the acrosome, head cap, and equatorial segment. (d): reaction in the anterior head cap of acrosome (e): posterior head cap. (f): in the neck (g): in part of acrosome and intermediate segment. (h): in the neck and intermediate segment. (i): predominant reaction in the anterior head cap. [MANCINI, GUTIERREZ, and FERNÁNDEZ COLLAZO; Fertil. Steril. 22, 475 (1971)]

Depending on the segment of the genital tract from which they are obtained, it seems clear that the four different sites of spermatozoa antigen-antibody interaction are: the acrosome, the postnuclear cap, the neck, and the intermediate segment or midpiece. The fact that acrosome and neck are reactive against most of the antibodies indicates that we are probably dealing with similar or different antigens that share common antigenicity. Testicular and epididymal spermatozoa may carry antigens in the acrosome related to those contained in the respective fluids, and these are mainly specific proteins, serum albumin, and lipoproteins. Other antigens attached to the remaining areas of the sperm cell may be produced in the accessory glands and related to those of the coating antigens (MANCINI et al., 1971).

The presence of specific "self" or "intrinsic" antigens in human spermatozoa, which do not originate in the seminal fluid, is still debatable. The observation that the washing of spermatozoa tends to weaken the staining in all the reactive areas is compatible with the extractability of the antigenic water-soluble fraction described above, while other antigens remain in the insoluble fraction as proved by immunoserologic methods. This difference points to low sensitivity or some other factors involved in the immunohistochemical techniques used. The presence of antigens of a different nature, such as serum proteins in sperm recovered from testis and in the ejaculate, indicates that perhaps they are coating the sperm, because they are contained in the seminal plasma and to a smaller extent, in seminiferous tubule fluid. In short, these results suggest that spermatozoa incorporate an increasing number of antigenic proteins in the head, neck and midpiece from the seminiferous tubules prior to ejaculation, and that this phenomenon may form a part of the complex process known as maturation of sperm.

Fluorescent Labeling. Other contributors to this topic (BROGAARD HANSEN and HJORT, 1971) have made use of the indirect immunofluorescent technique similar to that described above. Sera from children, blood donors, pregnant women, and wives from infertile couples were all tested. As a result four different staining patterns were observed in the following areas (a) the acrosome, its anterior part and the equatorial segment, (b) equatorial segment alone, (c) postnuclear area, and two fluorescent bands on the posterior third part of the head, (d) the tail, usually the main tail piece. Various combinations of these staining patterns were also seen, the most common one being the anterior zone of the acrosome and the equatorial segment. These findings, comparable to those involving homologous (FELTKAMP et al., 1965) or heterologous antisera (MANCINI et al., 1971), indicate that normal sera of adult subjects or of children can give positive results if used at low dilutions. This confirms the claim concerning the fluorescent staining of acrosome with normal sera of different species (EDWARDS, 1963). More intense staining reactions were encountered with a high frequency among sera from infertile patients, when used in dilutions ranging from $^1/_4 - ^1/_{16}$. With unfixed spermatozoa the reactions were weak and often uncharacteristic. After fixation with ethanol and acetone all four antigens were preserved, but after fixation with formalin the postnuclear antigen was not visible. The antigens in the equatorial segment and postnuclear region were destroyed at 60° C, and those in the front part of the acrosome and tail at 80° C. After trypsinization of the spermatozoa the reaction with the three antigens in the head disappeared. With rabbit antiserum to human spermatozoa, the fluorescence could be induced even after heating spermatozoa to 100° C, or treating them with trypsin. Absorption of human antisera with seminal plasma, human milk, liver, kidney or adrenal extract suggested an antigenic relationship between the antigen in the front part of the acrosome and the adrenal extract (BROGAARD HANSEN and HJORT, 1971).

By means of known antisera the occurrence of acrosome antigens in the individual spermatozoon has been investigated in ejaculates from 76 male partners of infertile couples. In ejaculates with a normal concentration of spermatozoa, the antigens were demonstrable in at least 50% of the spermatozoa, whereas samples with a low concentration showed a marked variation, the staining percentages ranging from 0% – 90% (BROGAARD HANSEN and HJORT, 1971). The occurrence of different antigens in the individual spermatozoon, in ejaculates from 13 highly fertile men and 29 men from infertile couples, has also been studied. The antigens were demonstrated by reaction with four human antisera and one rabbit antiserum. All semen samples contained the antigens, but the incidence of spermatozoa in which they could be shown varied considerably. The percentage in which the antigens were found was significantly correlated with the results of conventional semen analysis. The study suggested, moreover, that the best correlation exists between the percentage of spermatozoa reacting with antibodies against antigens in the sperm head and the percentage of motile spermatozoa. Antigens could, on the average, be demonstrated in a larger number of spermatozoa from fertile than from infertile men, which agrees with the finding that the results of semen analysis were also better in ejaculates from fertile subjects (BROGAARD HANSEN and REBBE, 1973).

False positive reactions due to the presence of ABO blood group antibodies could be disregarded, since the reactions were uncorrelated with the content of anti-A or anti-B in the sera, and independent of the ABO type of the sperm donors. Not all spermatozoa take up stain in the various reactions, even with the strongest sera; at most, two-thirds of them reveal the characteristic staining. Evidence in favour of the antibody nature of the serum factors was obtained using highly specific antisera against IgM and IgA. Antibodies against the front part of the acrosome seemed to be predominantly of the IgM class, whereas those reacting with the tail were exclusively of IgG class. Fractionation procedures with the same sera, by means of chromatography on DEAE cellulose or filtration through Sephadex G-200 and subsequent immunofluorescent testing of the concentrated fractions, revealed staining in full agreement with the immunohistochemical results (HJORT and BROGAARD HANSEN, 1971). Considered together, these observations indicate that a causal relationship exists between sera from infertile patients and the appearance of antibodies against different structures of the human spermatozoon. The hypothetical contention that the several antigenic reactive areas of the spermatozoon may respond to truly different antigenic entities remains a matter of speculation.

f) Blood Group Isoantigens

Another important class of antigenic substances for the human spermatozoon are the blood group isoantigens. By means of absorption techniques it has been possible to demonstrate the presence of A and B antigens in washed spermatozoa and in seminal plasma from subjects of the same blood groups (LANDSTEINER and LEVINE, 1926). At present there is still no agreement as to whether the spermatozoa of nonsecretors possess ABO antigens (POPIVANOV and VULCHANOV, 1962; EDWARDS et al., 1964; BOETT-CHER, 1965). The interest concerning the blood group and other isoantigens on spermatozoa is justified by the fact that gene segregation at meiosis could lead to the production of spermatozoa of a distinct phenotype, that is, types A and B from AB heterozygote, which would permit genetic studies on sperm samples. Some authors (EDWARDS et al., 1964) have attempted to show the presence of these isoantigens, using the mixed agglutination and mixed antiglobulin reaction. It was found that the spermatozoal membrane possesses "species-specific" antigens in common with red cells, probably corresponding to antigens of other tissue cells of the body. The A and B blood group isoantigens have been detected in the spermatozoa of secretors only. The presence of other isoantigens, such as M, N and Tja, has also been established; on the other hand, the sex-linked antigen Xga could not be seen in spermatozoa. Even before coming into contact with the seminal plasma, spermatozoa of secretor subjects have the opportunity to absorb ABO antigens, inasmuch as water-soluble antigens have been found in spermatocele fluid from a secretor subject and in epididymal spermatozoa (EDWARDS et al., 1964). Only traces of these antigens could be detected in the testis by absorption techniques (POPIVANOV et al., 1969), but they could not be demonstrated with corresponding antibodies labeled with fluorescein isothiocyanate (HOLBOROW et al., 1960). Presumably the seminal plasma is the main source of antigens for spermatozoa, perhaps chiefly the prostatic secretion (POPIVANOV et al., 1969).

As regards the biological effect of anti-blood group antisera on spermatozoa, it has been reported that exposure of spermatozoa to specific A or B antiserum does not produce any adverse effect on cell motility, although the specific antibody was noted to be absorbed by the sperm surface (SOLISH, 1969). With potent homologous immune sera of a high hemolytic activity, including group O serum, there were no changes in the immobilizing, agglutinating, and cytotoxic tests induced on ABO spermatozoa with the corresponding antibodies (FERNÁNDEZ COLLAZO and THIERER, 1972). However, it seems that some aspects of sperm metabolism, such as anaerobic glycolysis, could be affected by blood group antibodies (ACKERMAN, 1967; SOLISH, 1969). It is rather difficult to envisage what the biological significance of anti-ABO antibodies upon spermatozoa, bearing the respective antigens, might be, not only in the male reproductive tract but also in the female genital fluids. In this respect, it is interesting to record that in the cervical mucus of a group of sterile women the presence of these antibodies did not appear responsible for the immobilization, agglutination, and cytolysis of spermatozoa (PARISH and WARD, 1968).

g) Histocompatibility Antigens

In the course of the last few years there has been a discovery of marked interest concerning the biology of human spermatozoa. The histocompatibility antigens described in relation to animal spermatozoa have also been found in the human sperm cell (FELLOUS and DAUSSET, 1970). By means of the spermatotoxic test and using anti-HL-A typing sera from multiparous women, these authors have detected HL-A antigens on the membrane of human spermatozoa from healthy donors, previously typed for the same antigens by the lymphocytotoxic test. The typing sera corresponding to these antigens induced the lysis of only half the number of spermatozoa in samples from these heterozygous donors. In two other donors for whom family studies have detected homozygosity for the antigen HL-A2, the anti-HL-A2 serum induced a much higher degree of lysis of the spermatozoa. These differences in cytotoxicity from homozygous and heterozygous donors suggest the existence of two different populations of spermatozoa carrying on their membrane the expression of one haplotype of the HL-A loci. This is in full agreement with the presence of histocompatibility antigens on mouse spermatozoa and opens up an area for future study in infertility and homologous insemination. Recently HL-A "species" and "semen" antigens have been demonstrated on human spermatozoa by means of indirect immunofluorescence and immunoelectron-microscopy (KEREK et al., 1973). The observations indicated a homogenous, patchy, or occasionally discretely dotted distribution of HL-A antigens on the head and middle piece of the sperm cells, whereas "species" and "semen" antigens usually showed a discontinuous, patchy, or segmental distribution in the head and tail area.

3. Antigenicity of Human Seminal Plasma

Seminal plasma in the human, as in animals, is a mixture of secretions from the accessory glands of the reproductive tract and contains proteins specific for each of these organs, in addition to serum proteins. That humans are susceptible to sensitization by seminal plasma is supported by the unusual discovery of a woman showing a characteristic cutaneous allergic reaction following coitus. The responsible antigen was isolated by chromatography and identified as a protein with the structure and mobility of a beta-globulin (HALPERN et al., 1964).

a) Antigenic Components

The antigenic composition of seminal plasma has been studied by means of gel diffusion precipitation and immunoelectrophoresis, using antisera against serum proteins and several specific proteins contained in this fluid (KLOPSTOCK et al., 1963). Eleven components, 2 of them from the epididymis, 5 from the seminal vesicles, and 2 from the prostate gland, have been reported (LEITHOFF and GENKEL, 1964). A thorough study revealed a pattern of 9 components divided into 3 major groups; one of the leading lines corresponded to serum albumin, but only with partial antigenic relationship to it (HERRMANN and SCHIRREN, 1963). By immunodiffusion it was also demonstrated that human semen contains at least 16 antigens and the spermatozoa alone 7 antigens, 4 of the latter being common to seminal plasma (RAO et al., 1961). The number of specific proteins in seminal plasma has been shown to vary from 3 – 8, but in all cases the most prominent antigens showed beta-1 and beta-2 electrophoretic mobility (MISCHLER and REINECKE, 1966; SEARCY et al., 1964). Immunoelectrophoretic analysis of normal human seminal plasma with rabbit anti-human seminal plasma revealed 9 – 11 precipitin arcs. With human serum the antiserum showed 2 – 3 lines. Between seminal plasma and rabbit anti-human serum 2 or 3 lines were produced, a strong albumin line and 1 or 2 weak ones in the globulin region. It seems that seminal plasma albumin, although antigenically identical to serum albumin, is less apt to elicit antibodies. After absorption with lyophilized human serum, antiseminal plasma serum still produced 7 – 9 lines with seminal plasma. There is a discrepancy between the differences seen by agar and paper electrophoretic protein determinations and the constancy of the immunoelectrophoretic pattern (HEKMAN and RÜMKE, 1969).

By means of gel diffusion testing and careful selection of serum from several hyperimmunized rabbits, a maximum of 8 – 11 separate lines of precipitations has been described, and by immunoelectrophoresis 11 or 12 distinctive arcs were found (SHULMAN and BRONSON, 1969). An assembly of 4 major arcs or groups of arcs was seen and these were approximately the same short distance from the antibody trough but possessed widely different electrophoretic mobilities. In conclusion, there is a minimum number of reproducibly detectable components in seminal plasma equal to 12. Some of these components were shown to be related to serum proteins but only 1 of them was conspicuous in this respect and seemed to be antigenically identical to serum albumin. Fractionation by starch block electrophoresis has also been attempted and one major purified fraction was isolated, having a sedimentation coefficient of 1.0 S. This fraction was shown to be a component of the C group, probably of whole seminal plasma. In another report (HERRMANN and HERMANN, 1969) 8 components have been determined, including 2 aminopeptidases, several immunoglobulins, lactoferrin, a protease, and 2 acid phosphatases. Qualitative indications have also been provided on the presence of immunoglobulins in seminal plasma, particularly immunoglobulins IgG, A, and M, with variable concentrations in different samples and no clear-cut relationship to semen quality (BREHM and LACHNER, 1968).

b) Nature of Antigens

Apart from lactoferrin, which is a well-defined substance originating from the seminal vesicles but which behaves as a coating antigen for spermatozoa, other antigenic components have been studied. When human seminal plasma is treated with pronase, it loses 85% of its protein content, but the major antigens remain (AMANO and BEHRMAN, 1968). Of these, 2 seminal plasma specific antigens have been isolated by gel filtration on Sephadex-G-100 and characterized as mucoproteins with molecular weight of 40,000 and 20,000 respectively.

Failure to separate and characterize the coating antigen present in seminal plasma by routine precipitation procedures induced some authors (LIPPIELO et al., 1968) to use chromatographic methods. The results obtained led to the conclusion that the substance is a high molecular one and probably of mucoprotein nature, as shown by its behavior in chromatography with Sepharose 2B. These results were obtained from seminal plasma, in which the spermatozoa coating antigen had been concentrated free of material cross-reacting with antibodies against serum proteins, which are an important constituent of genital fluids.

A preliminary study of a trichloroacetic acid precipitable fraction from human seminal plasma has also been made. Studies of this fraction using Sephadex G-100 resulted in the isolation and characterization of 4 major glycoprotein entities, G1, G2, G3, and G4, on the basis of quantitative determination of amino acid composition, identification of sugar components, molecular weight, antigenicity, and immunoelectrophoresis (SCACCIATI, 1971, 1974). The technique used for the isolation of these glycopeptides did not involve the breakdown of covalent linkages. It is therefore probable that these products are actually present in the seminal plasma in their native state. The two glycopeptides G1 and G2 appear homogeneous by disc and cellogel electrophoresis, immunodiffusion, immunoelectrophoresis, and in the analytic ultracentrifuge. Proportionality between the molecular weights of these substances (average molecular weights of 10,800 and 10,400, respectively) and those corresponding to the mucoproteins mentioned above (AMANO and BEHRMAN, 1968; LI and BEHRMAN, 1970) has been noted, but the ratio between proteins and carbohydrates was much lower than the one present in the mucoproteins. Iron was absent and the carbohydrate content higher. Some similarity existed between the values of the sedimentation constant around S1.4 for both glycopeptides, and S1.5 for the three major compounds isolated from the seminal vesicle (SHULMAN and ORSINI, 1970). The amino acid composition was similar in both glycopeptides and only quantitative differences were observed (Table 8). The presence of sialic acid and the higher content of histidine in G1 make it likely that this

Table 8. Amino acid and carbohydrate composition of the two glycoproteins (G$_1$ and G$_2$) isolated from human seminal plasma. [SCACCIATI; Int. J. Fertil. 19, 211, (1975)]

Amino acid mg%	G$_1$ Residues/ 1000	G$_2$ residues	Carbohydrates	G$_1$ mg%	G$_2$
Aspartic acid	65.76	115.38	Total	86	86
Threoninie	209.10	88.75	Hexoses	90	90
Serine	141.65	82.84	Pentoses	0	0
Glutamic acid	80.94	147.92	Methyl-pentoses	0	0
Proline	11.80	2.95	Sialic acid	0.3	0.4
Glycine	64.08	115.38	Uronic acid	1.15	1.42
Alanine	69.13	100.59	Galactosamine	0.40	0.03
Valine	42.15	68.04	Glucosamine	0.20	0.06
Methionine	10.11	2.95	Chromatography	glu.-	glu.-
Isoleucine	33.72	32.54	of neutral sugars	gal.	gal.
Leucine	59.02	56.22			
Tyrosine	16.86	17.77		G$_1$	G$_2$
Phenylalanine	28.66	29.58		p. p. m.	p. p. m.
Histidine	82.63	29.58	Iron	0	0
Lysine	30.35	47.33			
Arginine	20.22	23.66			
Half-cystine	33.72	38.46			
Tryptophane	0.00	0.00			

chemical component, as proved in sensitized rabbits, is probably related to its high antigenicity. Corresponding antibodies showed a definite inhibition of motility of viable human ejaculated spermatozoa, sperm-agglutinating activity and a cytotoxic effect in the presence of complement. These antibodies can cross-react by immunodiffusion with repeatedly washed spermatozoa and attach selectively to the surface of the posterior part of the head and neck of the spermatozoa, as shown by the immunoperoxidase indirect technique (MANCINI et al., 1976).

Related to this study, 4 human seminal plasma specific antigens and 2 human seminal plasma milk common antigens have also been found (ISOJIMA, 1973). One of these antigens was identified as lactoferrin but the other is a different specific protein. Both seminal plasma-milk common antigens adhere to spermatozoa as coating antigens, as shown by an absorption technique using labeled antibodies to these antigens. By salting out, gel filtration, and DEAE cellulose chromatography, several fractions were obtained; one fraction contained 2 of the seminal plasma specific antigens and the other contained 1 of the seminal plasma-milk common antigens. An antibody against seminal-plasma antigen can immobilize spermatozoa in vitro, and it now seems probable that the immobilizing antibody found in the serum of a woman with unexplained sterility was not the antibody against seminal plasma-milk common antigen, but one against seminal-plasma specific antigen.

c) Origin of Antigens

To examine the origin and organ specificity of the antigens of seminal plasma, absorption experiments with several organ extracts were used (HEKMAN and RÜMKE, 1969). The 3 antigens originating in the prostate gland were organ-specific, since other organs or body fluids tested failed to give a reaction of identity. Two other antigens found in the seminal vesicle, were absent from other organs of the genital tract. Testis and epididymis reacted only weakly in double agar diffusion tests. Another weak line corresponded to a blood plasma component, against which the antiserum still contained antibodies after absorption with serum. The immunoelectrophoretic slides were stained for lipo- and glycoproteins and for a number of enzymes known to occur in seminal plasma. Strong glycoprotein staining was seen just anodic to the application well, in an ill-defined precipitate which stained faintly with amidoblack. It has been shown that milk and spleen contain one of the seminal vesicle antigens of human seminal plasma. This was confirmed in a double agar diffusion test, where the lines formed by anti-human seminal plasma with milk and spleen fused completely with one of the lines of seminal vesicle extract and seminal plasma. In a test arranged so that seminal plasma and milk could react with antiseminal plasma as well as with anti-human milk, only one continuous line was produced; the common antigen might be lactoferrin. As stated before, the presence of lactoferrin on the surface of spermatozoa has been confirmed by using antiseminal plasma serum previously absorbed with washed human spermatozoa. This antiserum was then tested with normal seminal plasma by immunoelectrophoresis; in the resulting pattern only the lactoferrin line had disappeared (HEKMAN and RÜMKE, 1969). Other authors claimed that one of the coating antigens is an ironbinding protein, sharing antigenic groups with lactoferrin but not with transferrin. They proposed to name it "scaferrin", although this distinction is only based on a difference in electrophoretic mobility (ROBERTS and BOETTCHER, 1969).

d) Cellular Immunity

Like human sperm, seminal plasma may elicit cellular immunity in guinea pigs, which can cross-react with spermatozoal antigens. The inhibition of macrophage migration and the effect of supernatant from sensitized lymph node cells incubated with seminal plasma, on the viability of motile spermatozoa and in the cytotoxic test, have been examined (MARCUS et al., 1973). The inhibition of migration of macrophages in the presence of seminal plasma is as intense as that obtained with human spermatozoa; they also show cross-reactivity. The cytotoxicity of supernatant from sensitized lymph node cells, as demonstrated by the Trypan blue penetration of spermatozoa, is higher than that induced by sensitization of guinea pigs with sperm. This cross-reaction of spermatozoa and seminal plasma in cellular immunity tests points again to common antigenicity between these two constituents of the male genital tract. If this phenomenon is not due to several antigens from seminal plasma coating the sperm, but to the existence of self "intrinsic" spermatozoal antigens, then it is something which deserves further investigation.

Another test for delayed hypersensitivity has been claimed as useful for the demonstration of cellular immunity reaction in humans. Blastoid transformation of sensitized peripheral leukocytes in vitro from self patient blood, in the presence of semen antigens, has been reported as positive in some cases of male sterility, whereas no positivity was found in a control group of presumably fertile men (EL-ALFI and BASSILI, 1970). In another group of infertile men no correlation was found between lymphocyte transformation and the presence of agglutinating or immobilizing antibodies and the sperm count (GORDON et al., 1971; MUNFORD et al., 1971). However, the lack of use of specific antigens from sperm or seminal plasma in the incubation with leukocytes make it difficult to interpret the results obtained, since the histocompatibility antigens, present in the donor semen, may interfere with the specific response of the leukocytes.

4. Antigenicity of Male Accessory Glands

There have been relatively few studies on human accessory glands. The interest of the investigators has centered mainly on the possible existence of separate characteristic antigens, in the glandular tissue and in the secretions. The induction of antibodies in the heterologous sensitization procedure, and also the potential damage developed by the accessory glands themselves, were major areas of study. This aspect is of great pathologic significance, in cases of disease localized in the prostate or seminal vesicle and the existence of concomitant humoral antibodies against spermatozoa, seminal plasma, and accessory glands. It was mentioned earlier (YANTORNO et al., 1971) that lesions of accessory glands have been induced in rabbits immunized with repeated doses of homologous or autologous seminal plasma (YANTORNO et al., 1973). Equally, it has been claimed that sensitization of animals with extracts of seminal vesicles can provoke inflammatory lesions of the gland (ORSINI and SHULMAN, 1971). However, so far, nobody has proved that immunization with any of the accessory glands can induce gonadal lesions and anti-testis antibodies.

As regards human accessory glands, our knowledge remains poor (SHULMAN, 1971). By agar immunodiffusion and a strong rabbit antibody against human seminal plasma, reactions against extracts of testis and epididymis were found to be weak. The most characteristic antigen present was lactoferrin, which was not demonstrable in the seminal plasma of patients with congenital absence of seminal vesicle (HEKMAN and RÜMKE, 1969).

The results of early investigations demonstrate that accessory glands, apart from their specific antigens, share one or two common autoantigens (FLOCKS et al., 1960). In addition to possessing several definitive tissue specific antigens, human prostatic fluid was shown to be a heterologous mixture of macromolecules as revealed by electrophoretic, ultracentrifugal, and enzymatic antigenic means. There have also been studies on proteases, phosphatases, and other enzymes (SHULMAN, 1971). A method for the detection of acid phosphatases by gel diffusion procedures using a specific staining method revealed 2 – 4 distinctive antigenic forms (SHULMAN and FERBER, 1966; SHULMAN and AHMED, 1971). A molecular weight of 84,000 and 470,000 for the major molecular forms has been claimed (MATTILA, 1969). Although auto- or homoantibodies to rabbit prostatic tissue can be produced in high titer, tissue damage or inflammation has never been found. However, claims have been made that serum from some patients with prostatic disease reacts with human prostatic extract, which implies that an autoimmune factor may be present (GRIMBLE, 1964). The possibility of injecting an anti-prostatic antibody fluid, in order to reach the recipient's prostate gland and perhaps influence beneficially a hypertrophied tissue, has also been explored (PEEL, 1968; MONCOURE *et al.,* 1968).

In an extensive study on the immunologic characterization of the human accessory glands, it was demonstrated that rabbit antibodies against saline extracts of prostate may cause agglutination of spermatozoa at higher titers than rabbit antibodies against extracts of testis, epididymis, and seminal vesicle. By immunodiffusion, prostate antiserum revealed 2 or 3 lines against seminal plasma and washed spermatozoa, and none with other organs, such as kidney, spleen or brain used as controls. Seminal vesicle antiserum also reacted against seminal plasma and spermatozoa but gave negative results with testis, kidney, and brain (BANDHAUER, 1966).

III. Antisperm Antibodies in Male Infertility

1. Clinical Findings

The pathologic significance, the incidence, and the possible implication of the antisperm and seminal plasma antibodies in cases of unexplained sterility will be described in this chapter.

Various immunoserologic and cellular immunity techniques have been used to explore the presence of antisperm antibodies in the serum and seminal plasma of male patients and in the blood and genital fluids of infertile women. The main purpose of such research was to find out whether there was a correlation between the occurrence of these antibodies, the impairment of spermatogenesis, and the systemic or local appearance of humoral or delayed hypersensitivity antibodies.

a) Spermagglutinating Antibodies

Early findings were concerned with spermagglutinins detectable in the serum of certain males (WILSON, 1954). In one instance, agglutination of the patient's own spermatozoa was due to the presence of autoantibodies in his semen. Sterility could be satisfactorily explained by the autoagglutination phenomenon; moreover, the agglutinated spermatozoa failed to penetrate the cervical mucus, whereas artificial insemination with donor semen was successfully performed in one of the patients. The other report (RÜMKE, 1954) dealt with 80 patients showing moderate or extreme oligozoospermia, two of whom seemed to have spermagglutinins in the serum with a high titer. In later studies using the same test for spermagglutinins, the sera of 2015 male partners of sterile couples were checked; approximately 3% seemed to have spermagglutinins in the serum with titers of $^1/_{32}$ or higher. This never occurred in the serum of 416 fertile men (RÜMKE and HELLINGA, 1959). There seemed to be a direct relationship between agglutination and the immobilization of spermatozoa induced by serum and other abnormalities, such as spontaneous agglutination and loss of motility of spermatozoa in the ejaculate of these patients. This correlation has often been observed when the serum spermagglutinin titer is high and agglutination in the ejaculate is strong and develops shortly after ejaculation. With low serum titers, seminal agglutination is either not present or sets in so slowly that it is not clearly visible within the first half hour; moreover, the clumps can be disrupted easily by mechanical agitation. Nevertheless, exceptions are not uncommon. Some patients have high titer spermagglutinins in the serum, without agglutination in the ejaculate, while others with low serum titers may show strong agglutination of the ejaculated spermatozoa (RÜMKE and HELLINGA, 1959).

When it became apparent that the main factor is the titer in the seminal fluid rather than in the serum, a series of 103 patients was examined and the serum as well as the seminal plasma were checked. In 94 cases the titer was 2 – 1024 times higher in serum than in seminal plasma; in 7, titers were equal and in 2 patients the seminal plasma titers were 8 and 64 times higher (RÜMKE, 1974). In some cases where the density and motility of the sperm in the ejaculate are near normal, autoagglutination being the only abnormal sign, sterility may be the direct outcome of the action of the autoantibody. This was evident from postcoital cervical mucus tests in a patient with total autoagglutination. In this case numerous motile, agglutinated spermatozoa were present in the vaginal secretion of the wife, whereas in the cervical mucus only a few immotile spermatozoa were detectable. In a retrospective study it was found that out of 137 patients with serum spermagglutinins and normal spermatogenesis, 30 became fathers; there was an inverse correlation between fertility and serum titers. In 22 cases where late re-examination of the serum was possible, with one exception, the fathers still had the same serum titers as were originally found (RÜMKE et al., 1973). As to the semen of patients having spermagglutinins in their serum, about a third had a normal sperm count and motility in the ejaculates; complete or partial autoagglutination was often observed in this group. Only a few patients showed no agglutination. Analysis of semen in one third of the patients showed low density, low motility, and often many epithelial cells or leukocytes; but morphology was nearly always normal. The remaining third suffered from azoospermia (RÜMKE, 1965).

The sera of 149 infertile women, 50 fertile women, and 227 pregnant women were tested with donor semen by the macroagglutination technique. The incidence of positive reactions varied with the quality of the donor semen specimens and a clear relationship between antibodies and infertility could not be demonstrated (NAKABAYASHI et al., 1961). An investigation dealing with ABO incompatibility, sperm autoagglutination and isoagglutination as immunologic factors of infertility has also been published (SCHWIMMER et al., 1967 a). It was found that (a) isoagglutinins occurred in 37.5% of 64 couples with primary unexplained infertility and in 50% of 32 couples with unexplained secondary infertility, as compared with 20% in control groups, (b) autoagglutination was not compatible with pregnancy, (c) circulating antisperm antibody fell to an undetectable level after 2 – 12 months of condom therapy, (d) in 48 prostitutes 72.9% positive titers were present to ejaculated sperm by the microagglutination test. The authors linked these findings with the decreased fertility of these women. With the help of a microagglutination technique, isoagglutination of spermatozoa in the sera of women with unexplained infertility has been detected. Preventing exposure of these women to their husband's ejaculate by abstinence, or by the use of condoms for 6 months, led to a fall of antibody titers to a serologically undetectable level, in 10 out of 13 women. After unprotected coitus timed with ovulation, 9 women became pregnant (FRANKLIN and DUKES, 1964). An extension of these studies over a population of 487 patients without demonstrable organic cause for infertility gave 25.0% positive results. A variety of different antibodies were found, including sperm immobilizing anti-

bodies and precipitins against components of the seminal plasma (DUKES and FRANK-
LIN, 1968). Following application of the macroagglutination test, it was concluded
that the presence of sperm agglutinins in the blood serum did not interfere with the
fertility of the individual, since in fertile men titers higher than $^1/_{32}$ have been found
(PHADKE and PADUKONE, 1964). In an investigation of 11 sterile couples, the male
partners had spontaneous agglutination of spermatozoa and sperm agglutinins in their
sera at higher titers. It was proposed that immunoagglutination of the spermatozoa
was probably the main cause of sterility in these marriages (FJALLBRANT, 1965).

In contrast with some of the above findings and utilizing a variety of techniques, it
was found that agglutination of the husbands' sperm by the wives' sera occurred in 13
out of 45 cases (29%), but in 10 the agglutinations were not due to antibodies in the
wife's serum, since control tubes also showed agglutination (ISRAELSTAM, 1969). Only
5% of the women with unexplained sterility had sperm agglutinins in the sera, when
spermatozoa from unrelated donors were used, but 14%, when those of the husbands
were used (TYLER et al. 1967). In a critical study (HANAFIAH et al., 1972) 11 husbands
who had positive sperm agglutination in their serum were examined. Four of
these were among 70 couples (5.6%) with no known cause for infertility, while the
other 7 were among 154 couples (4.5%) with a known cause. Five wives (45%) became pregnant without any treatment. The outcome of 8 out of 11 pregnancies was
normal delivery and no abortions, which shows that positive spermagglutination has
no effect on pregnancy.

As can be seen, the detection of agglutinating activity, although somewhat contra-
dictory to the results obtained, has been the most widely used test system in cases of
infertility. It depends on various circumstances, the most important being the source
of the semen. For instance, in a group of infertile couples, in one case the woman's serum was positive either with her husband's (autologous) or with a donor's (homologous) sperm. This kind of reactivity is characteristic in the majority of cases. In contrast, two other cases repeatedly showed a pattern of the woman's serum being completely negative with autologous sperm, but definitely positive with the homologous one.
The incidence of such a pattern is not known. Therefore the testing of the serum sample should be given adequate attention. It is important to test the serum from both
husband and wife, to use several semen specimens in repeated tests, and to employ two
or more procedures. Every semen sample should be evaluated with known positive and
negative sera and the results must be expressed quantitatively (SHULMAN, 1974). By
means of macro- and the microagglutination tests it was shown that the reaction is not
always specific for cases of unexplained sterility. In these instances it would seem that
the immobilization technique is the most specific method for testing antibodies that
impair the activity of spermatozoa (ISOJIMA et al., 1968).

b) Sperm Immobilizing Antibodies

In a group of 36 men having sperm antibodies, 15 of whom had fertile, and 21 sterile marriages, the sperm agglutinin titer and sperm immobilizing activity of the serum

were determined (FJALLBRANT, 1968 a). The penetration ability of the spermatozoa was investigated by means of postcoital tests and by two methods in which cervical mucus was used. The incidence of sperm antibody titers was higher in the sterile than in the fertile group. A negative correlation was found between the concentration of antibodies, particularly those with immobilizing activity, and the penetration of spermatozoa. The correlation between penetration ability and fertility was very good. It was concluded that sperm antibodies detected at high levels in the blood, particularly immobilizing antibodies, indicate a reduced penetration ability of spermatozoa and therefore low fertility in men. This investigation did not show whether the relationship between the level of sperm antibodies and sperm penetration ability is a causal one.

To investigate whether and to what extent spermatozoa from other men can be affected by sperm antibodies, semen samples from 6 fertile men were treated with rabbit antiseminal plasma serum and with serum from a man with sperm antibodies (FJALLBRANT, 1968 a). Semen aliquots from one donor were treated with different volumes of rabbit antiserum against seminal plasma, and spermatozoa from semen and spermatocele with serum from men with different concentrations of sperm antibodies in the blood. The penetration of the spermatozoa treated with antibody in cervical mucus was also investigated. Low concentrations of sperm antibodies reduced the sperm motility in mucus, and high concentrations reduced both the sperm motility in mucus and the extent of sperm penetration. When semen from 6 fertile donors was treated with rabbit antiserum against seminal plasma and with serum from a man with high sperm antibody concentration, the spermatozoa from all the donors were affected, but the penetrability of spermatozoa from ejaculates with high motility was less affected.

These results indicate that rabbit antibodies against human spermatozoa and seminal plasma, as well as those naturally occurring in males, can lower the extent of penetration of cervical mucus by spermatozoa. The degree of impairment depends on the antibody concentration and the intrinsic properties of the spermatozoa. The reduction of the ability of spermatozoa to penetrate mucus probably represents the mechanism whereby sperm antibodies may cause male sterility.

c) Cytotoxic Antibodies

Cytotoxic antibodies play a more important role in the development of experimental autoimmune orchitis than complement fixing and immobilizing antibodies. Much interest has centered on the possible existence of a cytotoxic antibody in cases of unexplained male sterility (HAMERLYNK and RÜMKE, 1968). In order to determine whether a normal spermatotoxic index could be found in cases where no antibodies could be expected, tests were made using the sera of 10 young fathers and 70 old nuns; in no case did the spermatotoxic index pass the statistical significance limit. As regards the serum of infertile males, a correlation was established between the spermatotoxic index and the presence and type of spermagglutinins. Studies on 35 sera with various spermagglutinin titers were tested and the existence of such a correlation could be demonstrated. The spermatotoxic index was found to be high in sera showing head-to-head agglutination, but those of the tip-to-tail type did not show spermatotoxic activity. In addition, some of the spermagglutinating sera had no spermatotoxic activity at all and conversely, the spermatotoxic index was found to be high in the absence of spermagglutinins. The correlation between quality and number of sperm and spermatotoxic antibodies was studied (HAMERLYNK and RÜMKE, 1968) in a group of 8 patients without, and another 6 with a high spermatotoxic index, both having comparable spermagglutinin titers. There was an indication of a correlation between the presence of spermatotoxic antibodies and oligozoospermia. Larger groups of patients are needed in order to establish whether this correlation really exists.

d) Immunofluorescent Antibodies

Apart from immunologic methods, the immunofluorescent test has also been applied to the study of sterility. The sperm microscopic agglutination and immobilization tests allow no distinction to be made between different antigen-antibody systems. It is only possible to distinguish between antibodies against different parts of spermatozoa, heads or tails. By means of immunofluorescent technique, a correlation was noted between the presence of spermagglutinins in the serum of 34 out of 77 male sterile patients and positive immunofluorescent results in the spermatozoa from donors (FELTKAMP et al., 1965). In another study with a group of similar patients, totally negative results have been reported (SOBBE et al., 1966). In men from infertile couples, positive results with immunofluorescent technique have been recorded in 74 sera out of 1340 (HAENSCH, 1969).

It is of interest that the higher frequency of positive immunofluorescent staining was seen in infertile patients and that a significant decrease in the number of positive reactions occurred when the serum dilution increased (FELTKAMP et al., 1965). The finding of high titers in some cases of pregnancy is of particular interest, since 2 out of 3 cases had been suffering from secondary infertility. The reaction with the sera of 2 children in a group of 82 was also uncorrelated to their sex and age. There was a predominance of strong staining reaction among women with unexplained infertility, as compared with those cases where the infertility might be explained. Immunofluorescence staining of the sperm head or midpiece with 10 out of 11 sera, which at the same time caused strong sperm agglutination, was detected. Positive reactions were obtained with sera from 46 out of 88 men over the age of 67, without spermagglutinins in the serum. Fluorescence of the tail was sometimes seen with sera showing no agglutination (FELTKAMP et al., 1965).

The sera from 9 infertile women with high titer of staining were tested by means of macroscopic sperm agglutination reaction, together with 9 sera from the same group and one control obtained from a man with spontaneous agglutination of the spermatozoa (HJORT and BROGAARD HANSEN, 1971). As only the latter case showed positive sperm agglutination, it seems that the immunologic system involved in the fluorescent test was not identical with that operating in the spermagglutinating test. Furthermore, there was a correlation between the spermatozoal concentration of a sperm sample and the ability to take up the fluorescent antibody. In general, ejaculates with a normal concentration exhibited staining of more than half the sperm. Ejaculates with a low sperm concentration showed a considerable number of spermatozoa having low staining. On the other hand, the immunofluorescent stainability of the spermatozoa showed no significant correlation with motility. The average number of stained spermatozoa was in all cases higher in the group with high motility than in those with poor motility; the lowest motility group showed a small number of stained spermatozoa. More precise studies are needed to decide whether motility may be correlated with the immunofluorescent test. Evidently, the immunofluorescent test offers the opportunity to verify the existence of a particular type of antisperm factor in infertility and probably of different antibodies depending on the site of the reaction in the spermatozoa, but the concentration of antibodies must also be taken into account (HJORT and BROGAARD HANSEN, 1971). So far, the occurrence of antisperm antibodies has been investigated by immunofluorescence to a limited extent, as compared with the spermagglutinating technique. Thus, the significance of these antibodies in relation to infertility is as yet uncertain.

e) Other Humoral Antibodies

By using the supernatant of frozen-thawed spermatozoa as an antigen, it has been possible to show the presence of sperm antibodies in the sera of infertile women by an hemagglutination technique (RAO and SADRI, 1959). The hemagglutination technique, using seminal plasma and washed spermatozoa as antigens, was also used to study the serum of 61 infertile men. Five men with positive titers to spermatozoa produced 2 pregnancies and 3 out of 6 infertile women with antibody titers became pregnant. It was deduced that serum factors demonstrated in this way did not interfere with normal reproduction (SOUTHHAM, 1963). The sera of 50 fertile and 45 infertile women were studied by the double agar immunodiffusion test, using as antigen the husband's seminal plasma. The incidence of positive precipitation reactions was 15% for infertile women (KATSH and KATSH, 1965).

In an extensive study of infertile couples using the hemagglutination technique and seminal plasma as antigen to detect antisperm antibodies, it was found that this serologic test gave a poor correlation with the microagglutination procedure and a low degree of reproducibility. Blood group isoantigens that may be present in seminal fluid can give false positive hemagglutination titers. Using the complement fixation test, preliminary studies show better correlation than the microagglutination test (SCHWIMMER et al., 1967 b).

Similar conclusions have been drawn from a study of 18 cases of unexplained female sterility, where 5 different immunologic reactions were applied, namely double agar diffusion, complement fixation, passive hemagglutination, spermagglutination, and indirect immunofluorescence; as antigens, seminal plasma and spermatozoa from their own husband's semen were employed. No antiseminal or spermatozoal antibodies were found in the sera of the women examined (COHEN, 1969).

2. Immunologic Pathogenesis

In the causal relationship between sperm antibodies and the development of unexplained cases of male sterility, as demonstrated by the use of humoral or cellular immunity techniques, two further points deserve consideration, which involve certain pathologic findings in the genital tract and the possible mechanism of autosensitization.

a) Pathologic Findings

In the case histories of 64 patients with spermagglutinin in the serum, data of significance were gonorrheal epididymitis, gonorrhea, herniorrhaphy in childhood, acute necrosis of testis after a surgical accident, minor surgery for spermatocele or fistula, mumps orchitis, inguinal abscess, leg ulcers, pulmonary tuberculosis, hemospermia, and syphilis. In about half the patients physical examination revealed abnormalities in the epididymis or vas deferens, often indicating that one or both of the efferent ducts were obstructed (RÜMKE, 1965).

In a study of the occurrence and etiology of sperm autoantibodies in the male, 1340 serum specimens of patients who consulted for sterility were examined, using the indirect immunofluorescent technique (HAENSCH, 1969). As stated above, inflammation of testes or epididymis and also trauma and dystopia of these organs may give rise to sperm fluorescent staining. In 26 patients the sperm count was normal and in another group of 15 patients an occlusive azoospermia was present. In 31 patients anomalies of location of testes and epididymis were noted. In these cases the frequent change of location, as for instance, in sliding testes always accompanied by mechanical irritation, must also be considered important. In more than half the patients with findings of sperm immunofluorescent antibodies, inflammation of testes or epididymis had occurred previously. Unspecific epididymitis, gonorrhea, tuberculosis, and orchitis following postpuberal epidemic parotitis can all initiate formation of antibodies. Quite frequently trauma to the testes is mentioned in the case history. Altogether, 19 out of 74 patients with sperm autoantibodies had experienced an inflammation or injury of the testes.

In another study (D'ALMEIDA et al., 1974), 88 serum samples from men seeking advice for sterility have been examined. This group comprised patients with oligoasthenospermia, spontaneous autoagglutination, epididymo-deferential anastomosis, aplasia of the deferent ducts, testicular traumatism and orchitis. Passive hemagglutination, immunofluorescence, cytotoxicity, mixed antiglobulin agglutination, complement fixation and double agar diffusion test were used. As a result it was observed that different techniques gave 22% positivity, 6% of which were positive in 3 of the reactions used. This global positivity corresponded to the autoagglutinins present in patients with previous history of retention and inflammation of the testis and epididymis. The authors assumed that positivity in all or in most of the tests must be considered a factor which diminishes fertility. A similar investigation has been carried out in a group of 489 patients who complained of infertility. The histories of these patients revealed inflammatory disease of testes, epididymis or ductus deferens; in some there was partial or total obstruction of vas deferens. Positive results in 14% were found, particularly demonstrable with spermagglutination and hemagglutination techniques (BANDHAUER, 1966). In a more recent study (ANDRADA et al., 1975) a group of 14 subjects was investigated who were suffering from acute or chronic mump orchitis. Complement fixation, hemagglutination, spermagglutination, sperm immobilization, and double agar diffusion tests were used; for delayed hypersensitivity, the skin test was performed using homologous sperm as antigen. Testicular biopsies were also obtained during the acute or chronic stage of the illness. Morphology of the testis showed that during the acute stage destruction of germinal cells and intense infiltration of polymorphonuclear leukocytes in the intertubular spaces and inside the seminiferous tubules occurred. This picture was replaced during the chronic stage by atrophy of germinative epithelium, peritubular fibrosis, and accumulation of mononuclear cells, mainly plasmocytes, lymphocytes, and macrophages around vessels in the subalbugineal and intertubular spaces. Except for sperm immobilization and spermagglutination, which appeared positive in the subacute and chronic stage, the serologic tests were negative at all stages of the disease. On the other hand, the skin test was consistently positive in the subacute and chronic phase, showing the typical histological picture of a delayed hypersensitivity reaction in about half the number of patients.

b) Mechanism of Autosensitization

Concerning the mechanism of autosensitization to sperm, the presence of damage in the testis or abnormalities in seminal spermatozoa of patients having sperm antibodies seems to be highly significant. In this respect, it has been repeatedly stated that the pathologic precedent of traumatism, inflammation or infection, which leads to a partial or total obstruction of different segments of the male genital tract, is coincident with a large percentage of positive results in immunoserologic techniques for antisperm antibodies. However, it must be remembered that appreciable numbers of positive results are obtained in sterile patients, with no apparent present or past signs of inflammation of the genital apparatus. According to several authors, obstruction in the efferent duct or inflammation of testis or epididymis due to different types of pathology, can lead to spermatostasis and consequently to extravasation of sperm or germinal cells into the interstitium of the epididymis or the testis. This is usually accompanied by infiltration of macrophages, lymphocytes, and plasma cells. The formation of a nonspecific granuloma in response to extravasation of sperm cells has been described in the epididymis (ZETTERGREN, 1958).

Sperm resorption may also take place in other conditions such as phagocytosis of sperm by leukocytes and especially macrophages in traumatic or gonorrheal epididymitis. This phenomenon is evident in the interstitium and lymph vessels of the epididymis and rete testis of cases of chronic epididymitis and is not rare in old people (WEGELIN, 1921; RÜMKE, 1972). Nonspecific granulomatous orchitis (CRUICKSHANK and STUART-SMITH, 1959), acute inflammatory diseases of genital tract (BANDHAUER, 1966), acute necrosis of testis (RÜMKE, 1965) and acute and chronic mump orchitis (ANDRÁDA et al., 1975) are illustrative examples of other conditions where destruction and extravasation of sperm is present. However, it has been claimed that in cases of obstructive azoospermia and after ligation of the vas deferens in man extravasation of sperm is uncommon. In these cases, phagocytosis of spermatozoa also occurring in physiologic conditions takes place in the lumen of the canaliculi of the epididymis in the basal epithelial cells where the sperm cells are metabolized; this lessens the possibility of an induction of a granuloma and consequent sensitization. In a review of 60 patients with spermatic granulomas, sperm was found in 19 instances in the lymph vessels in the vicinity of the granuloma or near spermatostasis (GLASSY and MOSTOLFI, 1956). In 6 out of 9 patients, besides inflammation, sperm phagocytosis, lysis, and agglutination of spermatozoa in the interstitium and tubuli of epididymis have been found (KING, 1955). Some cases of prostatitis have been reported to cause the formation of autoantisperm antibodies (FJALLBRANT and OBRANT, 1968). Recent studies on bilaterally vasectomized men demonstrated serum sperm agglutinating antibodies in 15 out of 27 men (55.5%) who returned for examination 1 year post-vasectomy. Sperm immobilizing antibodies were present in 11 cases (40.7%) and were encountered only when sperm agglutinating antibodies were present. Although the incidence of sperm antibodies in vasectomized men one year postoperatively remained comparable with that at six months, definite increases of sperm antibody titer have occurred in 5 men. Circulating sperm agglutinins were demonstrated in 19 out of 37 men (51.3%) at 6 weeks after bilateral vasectomy. Sperm immobilizing antibodies were present in 14 cases (37.8%), although 4 had no sperm agglutinins (ANSBACHER et al., 1972).

In animal experiments (ALEXANDER, 1973) absorption of spermatozoa after unilateral vasectomy affects differently the epididymis of the rhesus monkey and the rat. In the monkey, spermatozoa were ingested not by the epithelial cells but by macrophages. Agglutination of sperm was common in the lumen of efferent ducts of rhesus monkeys but not in rats; spermatozoa were broken down in the caput region of both of these animal species. Spermatocele on the vasectomized side was the rule in the rat, but the exception in the monkey. Some of these differences may have been due to the time lapse after vasectomy, which was up to seven years for the rhesus, but only eight months for the rat. It is also interesting to note that signs of active reabsorption of sperm were present on the unligated side.

These findings permit speculation that the site for autoimmunization of sperm is located in the connective tissue of the testis or of the accessory glands. Since normal spermatozoa, testicular or accessory gland tissue or secretion cannot induce "per se" antisperm antibodies unless an adjuvant is added, factors derived from local inflammation may serve to enhance by some unknown mechanism the autoantigenic properties of sperm cells. The formation of a granuloma, which would participate in the "processing" and promote the contact of the antigen with lymph vessels and the regional lymph nodes, would be the following step. This somewhat resembles the induction of autoallergic orchitis in one of the gonads of guinea pigs, when a thermal (RAPPAPORT et al., 1969; MANCINI et al., 1974) or a traumatic injury without the use of adjuvant (FAINBOIM et al., 1975) is inflicted on the contralateral testis. In such experiments, there is a remarkable correlation between cellular immunity and the presence of an intertubular granuloma in the injured testis which precedes the initiation of germinal cell damage in the contralateral testis.

An excessive immunizing dose of rat spermatozoa alone in isologous subcutaneous sensitization, without added adjuvant, induces the formation of spermagglutinins. Under these conditions no lesion of spermatogenesis is found in the testis (RÜMKE and TITUS, 1970). However, as some patients with obstruction of the efferents ducts with extravasation of sperm cells show no spermagglutinins in their serum, it is possible to speculate that other antibodies might be present or that factors other than extravasation of sperm are necessary, such as chronic excessive resorption of spermatozoa in the rete testis, efferent ducts or head of the epididymis, as well as great susceptibility of the local immune system (RÜMKE, 1965).

As in the case of experimental allergic orchitis, it is not yet known whether or not the circulating antibodies or the cellular immunity products must penetrate the seminiferous tubules to react with the germinal cells. For spermagglutinins this does not seem to be the case, since they have been often found in patients who had histologically normal testis. Conversely, cytotoxic antibodies are probably more important in this respect, as they have been seen in patients with abnormalities in the spermatogenic process, such as atrophy, disorganization, sloughing or varied degrees of arrest and in some cases mononuclear cell infiltration (HAMERLYNCK and RÜMKE, 1968). It is more difficult to envisage how these antibodies enter the seminal plasma to react with spermatozoa and reproduce *in vivo* the damaging effect that they can exert *in vitro*. In some cases the titer of spermagglutinins found in seminal plasma equals or is higher than that of the serum (RÜMKE, 1974) but no data are available on the presence of cytotoxic and immunofluorescent antibodies. Local production of antibodies by plasmocytes located in the connective tissue of the genital tract or diffused into and concentrated in the seminal plasma is another possibility. Evidence exists that IgA sperm antibodies are formed locally in the genital tract (COOMBS et al., 1973) and it has been claimed that IgG is also present in seminal plasma. In cases where the serum titer is much higher than in the seminal plasma, it can be assumed that serum antibodies are of the IgM type and would therefore not diffuse into the genital fluid.

Summarizing, one can say that although the concept of male sterility of immunologic origin may be accepted, it needs to be further examined in several aspects, particularly those referring to the presence of humoral antibodies and oligo- or azoospermia in the absence of damage to the testis.

Insufficient information on cellular immunity reactions, as well as lack of data on the use of more than a single sperm and seminal plasma antigen, do not allow a definite conclusion to be drawn on the correlation between autoimmunization to sperm antigens and infertility.

Conclusions

The purpose of this review has been to focus attention on the salient features of immune mechanisms related to the male reproductive process. To enable a better understanding of the role played by immunologic factors in testicular function and particularly in the induction of damage to the germinative epithelium, the purely experimental background as well as clinical findings have been discussed. The following are points which merit further consideration.

1. There are two antigenic systems in the male genital tract, one comprising testis, epididymis and the spermatozoa, and another which includes the prostate, seminal vesicle and seminal plasma. Antibodies against testis antigens react with epididymal sperm but not with accessory glands, whereas antiseminal plasma antibodies react with accessory glands and seminal sperm but only weakly with testis antigens. Testis antigens are carried by germinal cells, particularly spermatids and spermatozoa, and the acrosome appears as the predominant site of antigen accumulation. The existence of other nongerminal cell antigens, such as components of Leydig cells (androgens) and components of seminiferous tubule wall (basement membranes) and collagen, require further study. The maturation of spermatozoa is related to differences in antigenic potency, as testicular sperm cells are less immunogenic than ejaculated spermatozoa; an increasing number of different antigens coat the sperm cell during its transit along the genital tract. Glycoproteins, and more precisely glycopeptide molecules, are responsible for the antigenicity of the testis, sperm cell, and seminal plasma. More information is needed concerning the final purification and characterization of these antigens. This is also applicable to some other chemically related components present in sperm cells such as blood group isoantigens and histocompatibility antigens.

2. As a result of parenteral administration of homologous antigens alone, sperm humoral antibodies and weak testicular lesions may become detectable only after daily inoculations during several months. However, if a single intracutaneous injection of the same stimuli is combined with complete Freund's adjuvant, in an autologous or homologous immunization, the response involves not only humoral antibodies and cellular immunity but striking testicular damage and a dermal granuloma as well. With incomplete adjuvant testicular damage is not overt, but humoral antibodies of an anaphylactic type appear. To obtain an immunologic reaction and a unilateral testicular reaction without the addition of adjuvant, an inflammatory process subsequent to a thermal or traumatic injury must be induced in the contralateral testis; in such a case a typical granuloma can develop in the interstitial connective tissue of the injured gonad. The correlation between cellular immunity response and the presence of this

granuloma which precedes germinal cell damage in the contralateral testis is remarkable. An immunologic orchitis which includes a dermal granuloma is also evoked in the absence of adjuvants, by auto- or homologous intracutaneous inoculation with an homogenate prepared from thermally injured testes.

3. Under all these conditions the response known as allergic or immunologic orchitis (aspermatogenesis) is expressed by the development of progressive vacuolization of Sertoli cells, cellular and stage-specific lysis of germinal cells, and intertubular mononuclear cell infiltration accompanied by different types of humoral antibodies and cellular immunity, without damage in either the Leydig cells or the accessory glands. Unlike the testis antigens, seminal plasma or accessory gland antigens must be given in several doses with adjuvants to induce an equivalent testicular response.

4. Although the role of cellular immunity is generally accepted as predominant in the pathogenesis of this immunologic sterility, the simultaneous participation of humoral antibodies cannot be disregarded. Passive transference by intratesticular injection or parenteral administration in inbred receptors of lymph node cells or peritoneal macrophages from sensitized animals has been successful in reproducing the allergic orchitis. The antisperm serum injected by a systemic route requires the previous administration of complete adjuvant to obtain similar results. However, the direct intratesticular injection of immune serum alone is equally effective. Permeability of the rete testis is higher than that of the seminiferous tubules and the accessory glands, as regards the entry of antisperm antibodies which must interact with germinal cells or spermatozoa during transit. However, more information is needed concerning the presence of different immunoglobulin fractions and the development of cellular immunity in the various segments of the male genital tract.

5. In the human male, auto- or homoantigenic potency of the testis has been demonstrated. Selective alteration of the spermatogenic process, humoral antisperm antibodies, and cellular immunity were detected in response to the immunization with testis antigens added with adjuvant. Clinical studies of sterile patients indicate that pathologic precedent of traumatism, inflammation, or infection, which leads to a partial or total obstruction of any segment of the genital tract, is succeeded by a high percentage of positive results in immunologic tests for antisperm antibodies. Moreover, autoimmunization to sperm, as judged by positive results of sperm immobilization and agglutination, coincides more frequently with oligo- or azoospermia and abnormalities of accessory glands than with lesions of the testis. The presence of cytotoxic, immunofluorescent, and other humoral antibodies or cellular immunity have been insufficiently explored. Nevertheless, cytotoxic antibodies are probably more important in this respect, as they have been seen in patients with alterations of germinal epithelium and interstitial mononuclear cell infiltration.

6. It is then possible to postulate that immunologic factors may affect male fertility by impairment of the germinal epithelium and of seminal spermatozoa. In the latter case, antibodies must reach the seminal plasma via the accessory glands. This may lead to hypo- or aspermatogenesis when the testis is affected, or immobilization and agglutination of spermatozoa, if the interaction takes place in some other segment of the genital tract. It seems that antigens operate their release from germinal cells followed by

extravasation and resorption, more frequently seen in the epididymis than in the testis. The presence of sperm cell products in the adjacent connective tissue can induce inflammation and a specific granuloma. Presumably, local antibody production and the stimulation of the proximal lymph nodes can initiate a new release of antigens due to the interaction of germinal cells with antibodies; thus, a perpetuating circuit of self-destruction of germinal cells and seminal spermatozoa becomes operative. Since in this process more than one type of humoral antibodies and cellular immunity can develop, the absence of uniform criteria concerning the necessary testing procedures has interfered with progress in our understanding of the mechanism of sperm immunization. Therefore, further experimental as well as clinical studies are required in order to elucidate whether immunologic factors participate in the impairment of the spermatogenic process.

Acknowledgements

All my research works contained in this review have been carried out during the last fifteen years in the Immunology Laboratory of the Center for Studies on Reproduction, School of Medicine, University of Buenos Aires. They could not have been performed without the continuous financial support of the University of Buenos Aires, The Argentine Research Council (CONICET), The Ford Foundation and The Population Council, Inc., New York.

I wish to thank Drs. O. W. DAVIDSON, O. VILAR, M. NEMIROVSKY, O. BARQUET, A. ALONSO, R. MONASTIRSKY, M. P. BUENO, E. F. COLLAZO, A. BACHMANN, J. SCACCIATI, A. MAZZOLLI, C. BARRERA, L. FAINBOIM, A. C. SEIGUER, A. KIERSZENBAUM, B. DENDUCHIS and L. LUSTIG for their valuable collaboration, Drs. N. N. GÓNZALEZ and R. PUIG, Miss S. SERRATE, Mr. M. STEIN and Mr. M. AMBROSIO for their technical assistance and Mr. M. VARELA and Miss E. RUGERONI for their careful and efficient secretarial work.

References

ABLIN, R. J., SOANES, W. A., BRONSON, P. M.: Autoantibodies to rabbit testes as a consequence of "in situ" freezing. Folia Biol. (Praha) 17, 429 (1971).

ABREU, W. M., SANTA ROSA, G. L., LOBO, B. A.: Propiedades antigénicas de contenido da vesicula seminal do cobaio. An. Anat. brasil. 8, 39 (1963).

ACKERMAN, D. R.: Antibodies of the ABO system and the metabolism of human spermatozoa. Nature (Lond.) 213, 253 (1967).

ALEXANDER, N. J.: Ultrastructural changes in rat epididymis after vasectomy. Z. Zellforsch. 136, 177 (1973).

ALONSO, A., BUENO, M. P., SCACCIATI, J. M., GONZALEZ, N., MANCINI, R. E.: Serological reactivity of homologous and heterologous antitesticular antiserum against different guinea pig testicular antigens. Acta europ. Fertil. 1, 459 (1969).

AMANO, Y., BEHRMAN, S. J.: Immunochemical studies on human seminal plasma. II. Isolation and characterization of major antigens. Int. J. Fertil. 13, 61 (1968).

ANDRADA, J. A., ANDRADA, E. C., WITEBSKY, E.: Experimental auto-allergic orchitis in rhesus monkeys. Proc. Soc. exp. Biol. (N. Y.) 130, 1106 (1969).

ANDRADA, J. A., MENGONE, A., VAN DER WALDE, G., MANCINI, R. E.: Antisperm antibodies in mumps orchitis. Andrologia (1976) (in press).

ANSBACHER, R., KEUNG-YEUNG, K., WURSTER, J. C.: Sperm antibodies in vasectomized men. Fertil Steril 23, 640 (1972).

ARNASON, B. J., BRANISLAV, D., JANKOVIC, B. D., WAKSMAN, B. H., WENNERSTEN, C.: Suppressive effect of thymectomy at birth on reactions of delayed hypersensitivity. J. exp. Med. 116, 177 (1962).

ASHERSON, G. I., LOEWI, G.: The pressure transfer of delayed hypersensitivity in the guinea pig. Immunology 11, 277 (1966).

ATTARAN, S. E., HODGES, C. V., CRARY, L. S., VANGA DER, G. C., LAWSON, R. K. ELLIS, L. R.: Homotransplants of the testis. J. Urol. 95, 387 (1966).

BANDHAUER, K.: Immunoreaktionen bei Fertilitätsstörungen des Mannes. Urol. int. (Basel) 21, 247 (1966).

BARNES, A. D.: A quantitative comparison study of immunizing ability of different tissues. N. Y. Acad. Sc. 120, 237 (1964).

BARRERA, C., MAZZOLLI, A. B., MANCINI, R. E.: Cytophilic activity in experimental immunological orchitis in guinea pigs. Fertil Steril (1976) (in press).

BARTH, R. F., RUSSELL, P. S.: The antigenic specificity of spermatozoa. I. An immunofluorescent study of the histocompatibility antigens of mouse sperm. J. Immunol. 93, 13 (1964).

BASKIN, M. J.: Temporary sterilization by the injection of human spermatozoa (a preliminary report) Amer. J. Obstet. Gynec. 24, 892 (1932).

BAUM, J.: Reaction of guinea pig spermatozoa with homologous antibody. Lancet 1959 I, 810.

BEISER, S. M., ERLANGER, B. F., AGATE, F. J. Jr., LIEBERMANN, S.: Antigenicity of steroid-protein conjugates. Science 129, 564 (1959).

BERKEN, A., BENACERRAF, B.: Properties of antibodies cytophilic for macrophages. J. exp. Med. 123, 119 (1966).

BISHOP, D. W.: Aspermatogenesis induced by testicular antigen uncombined with adjuvants. Proc. Soc. exp. Biol. Med. (N. Y.) **107**, 116 (1961).

BISHOP, D. W.: Sorbitol dehydrogenase. Enzymic antigen and assay for induced aspermatogenesis. In: International Convocation on Immunology p. 384: ROSE, N. R. and MILGROM, F. (eds.), Basel: KARGER, 1969.

BISHOP, D. W.: Immunological responses of the testis. In: The Testis, Vol. III. p. 41, JOHNSON, A. D., GOMES, W. R. and VANDEMARK, N. L. (eds.), New York: Academic Press 1970.

BISHOP D. W., CARLSON, G. L.: Immunologically induced aspermatogenesis in guinea pigs. Ann. N. Y. Acad. Sci. **124**, 247 (1965).

BISHOP, D. W., NARBAITZ, R., LESSOF, M.: Induced aspermatogenesis in adult guinea pigs injected with testicular antigen and adjuvant in neonatal stages. Develop. Biol. **3**, 444 (1961).

BOETTCHER, B.: Human ABO blood group antigens on spermatozoa from secretors and non-secretors. J. Reprod. Fertil. **9**, 267 (1965).

BOETTCHER, B., KAY, D. J.: Fractionation of a human spermagglutinating serum. Nature (Lond.) **223**, 737 (1969).

BOUGHTON, B., SCHILD, S.: Transfer of delayed hypersensitivity by lymph node cells in testis autosensitization. Immunology **5**, 222 (1962).

BOUGHTON, B., SPECTOR, W. G.: Autoimmune testicular lesions induced by injury to the contralateral testis and intradermal injection of adjuvant. J. Path. Bact. **86**, 69 (1963).

BOYDEN, S. V., SORKIN, E.: The absorption of antigen by spleen cells previously treated with antiserum "in vitro" – Some further experiments. Immunology **4**, 244 (1961).

BRATANOV, K., DIKOV, V., TORNYOV, A., PAVLOVA, S.: Study on the antigenic properties of ram's semen. In: Proc. IInd. int. Symp. on Immunology of Reproduction p. 180. BRATANOV, K., EDWARDS, R. G., VULCHANOV, V. H., DIKOV, V., SOMLEV, B. (eds.). Bulgarian Academy of Sciences Press 1973.

BREHM, G., LACHNER, H.: Quantitative Immunoglobulinbestimmungen im Seminalplasma. Klin. Wschr. **46**, 902 (1968).

BROGAARD, HANSEN, K., HJORT, T.: Immunofluorescent studies on human spermatozoa. II. Characterization of spermatozoal antigens and their occurence in spermatozoa from the male partners of infertile couples. Clin. exp. Immunol. **9**, 21 (1971).

BROGAARD HANSEN, K., REBBE, H.: Immunofluorescent studies on human spermatozoa. Int. J. Fertil. **18**, 101 (1973).

BROWN, P. C., DORLING, J., GLYNN, L. E.: Ultrastructural changes in experimental allergic orchitis in guinea pigs. J. Pathol. **106**, 229 (1972).

BROWN, P. C., GLYNN, L. E., HOLBOROW, E. J.: The pathogenesis of experimental allergic orchitis in guinea pigs. J. Path. Bact. **86**, 505 (1963).

BROWN, P. C., GLYNN, L. E., HOLBOROW, E. J.: The dual necessity for delayed hypersensitivity and circulating antibodies in the pathogenesis of experimental allergic orchitis in guinea pigs. Immunology **13**, 307 (1967).

BROWN, P. C., HOLBOROW, E. J., GLYNN, L. E.: The aspermatogenic antigen in experimental allergic orchitis in guinea pigs. Immunology **9**, 255 (1965).

CHANG, M. C.: The effects of serum on spermatozoa. J. Gen. Physiol. **30**, 321 (1947).

CHERNYSHOV, V. P., PODOPLELOV, I. L.: Immunobiological studies of the prostate gland and spermatozoa. In: Proc. IInd. Int. Symp. on Immunology of Reproduction, p. 241. BRATANOV, K., EDWARDS, R. G., VULCHANOV, V. H., DIKOV, V., SOMLEV, B. (eds.). Bulgarian Academy of Sciences Press 1973.

CHEVIAKOFF, S., CALAMERA, J. C., MORGENFELD, M., MANCINI, R. E.: Recovery of spermatogenesis in patients with lymphoma after treatment with Chlorambucil. J. Reprod. Fertil. **33**, 155 (1973).

CHUTNÁ, J., RYCHLIKOVA, M.: A study of the biological effectiveness of antibodies in the development and prevention of experimental autoimmune aspermatogenesis. Folia biol. **10**, 188 (1964 a).

CHUTNÁ, J., RYCHLIKOVA, M.: Prevention and suppression of experimental aspermatogenesis in adult guinea pigs. Folia biol. 10, 177 (1964 b).

CLEMONT, Y., GLEGG, R. E., LEBLOND, C. P.: Presence of carbohydrates in the acrosome of the guinea pig spermatozoa. Exp. cell Res. 8, 453 (1955).

COHEN, J.: Immunological factors and unexplained sterility. Acta europ. Fertil. 1, 193 (1969).

COOMBS, R. R. A., RÜMKE, P., EDWARDS, R. G.: Immunoglobulin classes reactive with spermatozoa in the serum and seminal plasma of vasectomized and infertile men. In: Proc. IInd. Int. Symp. on Immunology of Reproduction, p. 354. BRATANOV K., EDWARDS, R. G. VULCHANOV, V. H., DIKOV, V., SOMLEV, B.(eds.), Bulgarian Academy of Science Press 1973.

CRUICKSHANK, B., STUART-SMITH, D. A.: Orchitis associated with sperm-agglutinating antibodies. Lancet 1959 I, 708.

D'ALMEIDA, M., BELAISCH, J., EYQUEM, A., GUILLON, G., PALMER, R.: cit in: COHEN, J.: Immunological factors and unexplained sterility. Acta europ. Fertil. 1, 193 (1969).

D'ALMEIDA, M., KLEIN, R., PERONI, M.: Antisperm autoimmunity and male sterility. Acta europ. Fertil. 5, 241 (1974).

DELAUNAY, A., VOISIN, G. A.: Sur des lésions testiculaires provoquées chez le cobaye et chez le rat par l'endotoxine typhique. C. R. Soc. Biol. (Paris) 234, 168 (1952).

DENDUCHIS, B., LUSTIG, L., GONZÁLES, N. N., MANCINI, R. E.: Isolation and chemical characterization of seminiferous tubule basement membrane. Biol. Reprod. 13, 274 (1975).

DONDERO, F., ISIDORI, A.: Autoimmunisation antitesticulaire chez l'homme. Anns. Endocr. (Paris) 33, 417 (1972).

DUKES, C. D., FRANKLIN, R. R.: Sperm agglutinins and human female infertility. Fertil. Steril. 19, 263 (1968).

EDWARDS, R. G.: Complement fixing activity of normal rabbit serum with rabbit spermatozoa and seminal plasma. J. Reprod. Fertil. 1, 268 (1960).

EDWARDS, R. G.: The antigenicity of mammalian spermatozoa and its relationship to induced infertility. In: Proc. VIIth. Inter. Conf. Planned Parenthood p. 539., Excerpta Medica Inter. Cong. Series No. 72, 1963.

EDWARDS, R. G., FERGUSON, L. C., COOMBS, R. R. A.: Blood group antigens on human spermatozoa. J. Reprod. Fertil. 7, 153 (1964).

EL-ALFI, O. S., BASSILI, F.: Immunological spermatogenesis in man. I. Blastoid transformation of lymphocytes in response to seminal antigen in cases of non-obstructive azoospermia. J. Reprod. Fertil. 21, 23 (1970).

ERICKSON, R. P.: Alternative modes of detection of H-2 antigens on mouse spermatozoa. In: Proc. Inter. Symp. on Genetics of the Spermatozoon p. 191. BEATTY, R. A., and GLUECKSOHN-WAELSCH, S. (eds.) Copenhagen: Bogtrykkeriet Forum 1971.

EVREV, T., ZHIVKOV, R., POPIVANOV, R., KEHAYOV, I., PODOPLELOV, I., GLYNSKY, A., KRUYKOV, V. G.: Immunological studies on some isoenzymes of testis and spermatozoa. In: Proc. IInd. Int. Symp. on Immunology of Reproduction p. 228. BRATANOV, K., EDWARDS, R. G., VULCHANOV, V. H., DIKOV, V., SOMLEV, B. (eds.), Bulgarian Academy of Science Press 1973.

EYQUEM, A., KRIEG, H.: Experimental autosensitization of the testis. Ann. N. Y. Acad. Sci. 124, 270 (1965).

FAINBOIM, L., BARRERA, C., MANCINI, R. E.: Effect of unilateral traumatic orchitis on the contralateral gonad. Andrologia (1976) (in press).

FAINBOIM, L., STEIN, M., CERRATE, S., MANCINI, R. E.: Passive homologous transfer of immunologic orchitis to guinea pigs by RNA preparation extracted from lymph nodes of sensitized animals. p. 197 Proc. Inter. Sympos. on Immunology of Reproduction, Varna. Bulgarian Academy of Science Press 1975.

FARNUM, C. G.: The biologic test for semen. J. A. M. A. 37, 1721 (1901).

FAWCETT, D. W., LEAK, L. V., HEIDGER, P. M.: Electron microscopic observations on the structural components of the blood-testis barrier. J. Reprod. Fertil. Suppl. 10, 105 (1970).

FELLOUS, M., DAUSSET, J.: Probable haploid expression of HL-A antigens on human spermatozoa. Nature (Lond.) **225**, 191 (1970).

FELTKAMP. T. E. W., KRUYFF, K., LADIGES, N. C. J. J., RÜMKE, P.: Autospermagglutinins immunofluorescent studies. Ann. N. Y. Acad. Sci. **124**, 702 (1965).

FERNÁNDEZ COLLAZO, E., THIERER, E.: Action of ABO antisera on human spermatozoa. Fertil. Steril. **23**, 376 (1972).

FERNÁNDEZ COLLAZO, E., THIERER, E., MANCINI, R. E.: Immunologic and testicular response in guinea pigs after unilaterial thermal orchitis. J. Allergy and Clin. Immunol. **49**, 167 (1972).

FISHMAN, M., ADLER, F., RICE., G. S.: Macrophage RNA in the *in vitro* immune response to phage. In: RNA in the immune response. FRIEDMAN, H. (ed). Ann. N. Y. Acad. Sci. **207**, 73 (1973).

FJALLBRANT, B.: Immunoagglutination of sperm in cases of sterility. Acta, obstet. gynec. scand. **44**, 474 (1965).

FJALLBRANT, B.: Sperm agglutinins in sterile and fertile men. Acta obstet. gynec. scand. **47**, 89 (1968 a).

FJALLBRANT, B.: Studies on sera from men with sperm antibodies. Acta obstet. gynec. scand. **48**, 131 (1968 b).

FJALBRANT, B., OBRANT, O.: Clinical and seminal findings in men with sperm antibodies. Acta obstet. gynec. scand. **47**, 151 (1968).

FLOCKS, R. H., URICH, V. C., PATEL, C. A., OPITZ, J. M.: Studies on the antigenic properties of prostatic tissue. Int. J. Urol. (Baltimore) **84**, 134 (1960).

FRANKLIN, R. R., DUKES, C. D.: Further studies on spermagglutinating antibody and unexplained infertility. J. Amer. med. Ass. **190**, 682 (1964).

FREUND, J., LIPTON, M. M., THOMPSON, G. E.: Aspermatogenesis in guinea pig induced by testicular tissue and adjuvant. J. exp. Med. **97**, 711 (1953).

FREUND, J., LIPTON, M. M., THOMPSON, G. E.: Impairment of spermatogenesis in the rat after cutaneous injection of testicular suspension with complete adjuvant. Proc. Soc. exp. Biol. Med. (N. Y.) **87**, 408 (1954).

FREUND, J., THOMPSON, G. E., LIPTON, M. M.: Aspermatogenesis, anaphylaxis and cutaneous sensitization induced in guinea pigs by homologous testicular extract. J. exp. Med. **101**, 591 (1955).

GEORGE, M., VAUGHAN, J. H.: "In vitro" cell migration as a model for delayed hypersensitivity. Proc. Soc. exp. Biol. Med. **111**, 514 (1962).

GLASSY, F. J., MOSTOFI, F. K.: Spermatic granulomas of the epididymis. Am. J. clin. Path. **26**, 1303 (1956).

GORDON, H. L., BARSALES, P. B., WESTERMAN, E. L., MUNFORD, D. M.: Microlymphocyte transformation studies with seminal antigens. II. Observations in male patients with sperm agglutinating antibodies. J. Urol. **105**, 863 (1971).

GRANGER, G. A.: Mechanisms of lymphocyte- induced cell and tissue destruction in vitro. Amer. J. Pathol. **60**, 469 (1970).

GREEN, H., SILVERBLATT, F.: Effect of antibody and complement on volume control in an ascites tumor cell. Nature **186**, 646 (1960).

GRIMBLE, A.: Auto-immunity to prostate antigen in rheumatic diseases. J. clin. Path. **17**, 264 (1964).

GUYER, M. P.: Studies on cytolysins. III. Experiments with spermatoxins. J. exp. Zool. **35**, 207 (1922).

HAENSCH, R.: Fluorescenzimmunologische Spermienautoantikörperbefunde bei männlichen Fertilitatsstörungen. Arch. Gynak. **208**, 91 (1969).

HALPERN, B., KY, N., ROBERT, B.: Etude immunologique d'un cas exceptionnel de sensibilisation spontanée au semen humain. C. R. Acad. Sc. Paris **259**, 2025 (1964).

HAMERLYNCK, J. V., RÜMKE, P.: Spermatotoxic antibodies in man. J. Reprod. Fertil. **17**, 191 (1968).

HANAFIAH, M. J., EPSTEIN, J. A., SOBRERO, A. J.: Sperm-agglutinating antibodies in 236 infertile couples. Fertil. Steril. 23, 493 (1972).

HARGIS, B. J., MALKIEL, S., BERKELHAMMER, J.: Immunologically induced aspermatogenesis in the white mouse. J. Immunol. 101, 374 (1968).

HATHAWAY, R. R., HARTREE, E. F.: Observations on the mammalian acrosome; experimental removal of acrosome from ram and bull spermatozoa. J. Reprod. Fertil. 5, 225 (1963).

HEKMAN, A., RÜMKE, P.: The antigens of human seminal plasma. Fertil. Steril. 20, 312 (1969).

HENLE, W.: The specificity of some mammalian spermatozoa. J. Immunol. 34, 324 (1938).

HENLE, W., HENLE, G., CHAMBER, L. A.: Studies on the antigenic structure of some mammalian spermatozoa. J. exp. Med. 68, 335 (1938).

HERRMANN, W. P., HERMANN, G.: Immunoelectrophoretic and chromatographic demonstration of IgG, IgA and fragments of γ-globulin in the human seminal fluid. Int. J. Fertil. 14, 211 (1969).

HERMANN, W. P., SCHIRREN, C.: Immunoelektrophoretische Untersuchungen des menschlichen Spermaplasma. Z. Haut- u. Geschl. Kr. 34, 134 (1963).

HJORT, T., BROGAARD HANSEN, K.: Immunofluorescent studies on human spermatozoa. I. The detection of different spermatozoal antibodies and their occurrence in normal and infertile women. Clin. exp. Immunol. 8, 9 (1971).

HOLBOROW, E. J., BROWN, P. C., GLYNN, L. E., HAWES, M. D., GRESHAM, D. A., O'BRIEN, T. F., COOMBS, R. R. A.: The distribution of the blood group antigens in human tissues. Brit. J. Exp. Pathol. 41, 430 (1960).

HUNTER, A. G.: Differentiation of rabbit sperm antigens from those of seminal plasma. J. Reprod. Fertil. 20, 143 (1969).

ISOJIMA, S.: Antibodies against spermatozoa found in women and corresponding antigens in human semen. Proc. Ist. Inter. Cong. on Immunology in Obstetrics and Gynecology, p. 5 CENTARO, A., CARRETTI, N., and ADDISON, G. M. (eds.). Inter. Cong. Series No. 281. Amsterdam: Excerpta Medica, 1973.

ISOJIMA, S., STEPUS, S.: Antigenicity of guinea pig testis and ovary. Int. Arch. Allergy 15, 350 (1959).

ISOJIMA, S., STEPUS, S., ASHITAKA, Y.: Immunologic analysis of sperm immobilizing factor found in sera of women with unexplained sterility. Amer. J. Obstet. Gynec. 101, 677 (1968).

ISOJIMA, S., TIEN, SHUN LI: Stepwise appearance of sperm specific antigens in rats and their disappearance after fertilization. Fertil. Steril. 19, 999 (1968).

ISRAELSTAM, D. M.: The incidence of sperm-agglutinating in the serum of infertile women. Fertil. Steril. 20, 275 (1969).

JACKSON, H., FOX, B. W., CRAIG, A. W.: Antifertility substances and their assessment in the male rodent. J. Reprod. Fertil. 2, 447 (1961).

JANKOVIC, B. D., FLAX, M. H.: Alterations in the development of experimental allergic thyroiditis induced by injection of homologous thyroid extract. J. Immunol. 90, 178 (1963).

JOHNSON, M. H.: Characterization of a natural antibody in normal guinea pig serum reacting with homologous spermatozoa. J. Reprod. Fertil. 16, 503 (1968).

JOHNSON, M. H.: An immunological barrier in the guinea pig testis. J. Pathol. 101, 129 (1970 a).

JOHNSON, M. H.: Changes in the blood testis barrier of the guinea pig in relation to histological damage following iso-immunization with testis. J. Reprod. Fertil. 22, 119 (1970 b).

JOHNSON, M. H., SETCHELL, B. P.: Protein and immunoglobulin content of rete testis fluid of rams. J. Reprod. Fertil. 17, 403 (1968).

KANTOR, G. L., DIXON, F. J.: Transfer of experimental allergic orchitis with peritoneal exudate cells. J. Immunol. 108, 329 (1972).

KARUSH, F., EISEN, H. N.: A theory of delayed hypersensitivity. Science 136, 1032 (1962).

KATSH, S.: Immunology, fertility and infertility; a historical review. Amer. J. Obstet. Gynec. 77, 946 (1959).

KATSH, S.: Localization and identification of aspermatogenic factor in guinea pig testicles. Int. Arch. Allergy (Basel) 16, 241 (1960 a).

KATSH, S.: The anaphylactogenicity of testicular hyaluronidase and a species difference in testicular hyaluronidase demonstrated by isolated organ anaphylaxis. Int. Arch. Allergy Appl. Immunol. 17, 70 (1960 b).

KATSH, S.: Antigenicity of human testis. J. Urol. (Baltimore) 87, 896 (1960 c).

KATSH, S., AGUIRRE, A. R., LEAVER, F. W., KATSH, G. F.: Purification and partial characterization of aspermatogenic antigen. Fertil. Steril. 9, 644 (1972).

KATSH, S., CROWLE, A. J., KATSH, G. F.: Non-mycobacterial adjuvant which mediates experimental aspermatogenesis. Nature (Lond.) 212, 1486 (1966).

KATSH, S., DUNCAN, G. W.: Pituitary gonadotropin content of aspermatogenic guinea pigs. Proc. Soc. exp. Biol. Med. 127, 470 (1968).

KATSH, S., KATSH, G. F.: Antigenicity of spermatozoa. Fertil. Steril. 12, 522 (1961).

KATSH, S., KATSH, G. F.: Perspectives in immunological control for reproduction; past, present and future. Pacific Med. Surg. 73, 28 (1965).

KATSH, S., KATSH, G. F.: Enzyme inactivation of aspermatogenic antigen. Nature 212, 1486 (1966).

KENNEDY, W. P.: The production of spermatotoxins. Quart. J. exp. Physiol. 14, 179 (1924).

KERÉK, G., BIBERFELD, P., AFZELIUS, B. A.: Demonstration of HL-A antigens, "Species" and " Semen"-specific antigens on human spermatozoa. Int. J. Fertil. 18, 145 (1973).

KIBRICK, S., BELDING, D. L., MERRILL, B.: Methods for the detection of antibodies against mammalian spermatozoa. II A gelatin agglutination test. Fertil. Steril. 3, 430 (1952).

KIERSZENBAUM, A. L., MANCINI, R. E.: Structural changes manifested by Sertoli cells during experimental allergic orchitis in guinea pigs. J. Reprod. Fertil. 33, 119 (1973).

KING, E. S. J.: Spermatozoal invasion of epididymis. J. Path. Bact. 70, 459 (1955).

KIRKPATRICK, C. H., KATSH, S.: Aminoacid content of antispermatogenic antigen. Nature (Lond.) 201, 197 (1964).

KLOPSTOCK, A., HAAS, R., RIMON, A.: Immunoelectrophoretic analysis of seminal plasma. Fertil. Steril. 14, 530 (1963).

KOLK, A. H. J., SAMUEL, T., RÜMKE, P.: Autoantigens of human spermatozoa. I. Solubilization of a new auto-antigen detected on swollen spermheads. J. Clin. Exp. Immunol. 16, 63 (1974).

KORMANO, M.: Penetration of intravenous trypan blue into the rat testis and epididymis. Acta Histochem. 30, 133 (1968).

LACOMBE, F. P., TEXEIRA, C. A.: A anespermatogenese produzida em coelhos por injecoes de homogenatos de espermatozoides e de testiculos de cobaios con adjuvante incompleto. An. Col. Anat. Brasileira 8, 39 (1963).

LANDSTEINER, K.: Zur Kenntnis der spezifisch auf Blutkörperchen wirkenden Sera. Zentralbl. Bakteriol. Parasitenk. 25, 546 (1899).

LANDSTEINER, K., LEVINE, P.: On group specific substances in human spermatozoa. J. Immunol. 12, 415 (1926).

LAURENCE, K. A., CARPUK, B. A., PERLBACHS, M.: Transfer of testicular lesions by leukocytes from testis-immunized rats. Int. J. Fertil. 10, 13 (1965).

LAWRENCE, H. S.: Transfer factor and cellular immunity. Hospital Practice 4, 40 (1969).

LAWRENCE, H. S., VALENTINE, F. T.: Transfer factor and other mediators of cellular immunity. Amer. J. Pathol. 60, 437 (1970).

LE BOUTELIER, P., TOULET, F., VOISIN, G. A.: Etude ultrastructurale des lésions specifiquement induites par l'auto-anticorps anti-auto-antigene T sur les spermatozoides épididymaires de cobaye. C. R.Acad. Sc. Paris 276, 1509 (1973).

LEE, S., TUNG, K. S., ORLOFF, M. J.: Testicular transplantation in the rat. Trans. Proc. 3, 586 (1971).

LEITHOFF, H., GENKEL, U.: Die Herkunft der organspezifischen Proteine des menschlichen Samenplasmas. Med. Welt. (Berl.) 3, 2073 (1964).

Lerner, R. D., Dixon, F. J.: Transfer of ovine experimental allergic glomerulonephritis (E. A. G.) with serum. J. exp. Med. 124, 431 (1966).

Levine, S., Sowinski, R.: Allergic inflammation, infarction and induced localization in the testis. Amer. J. Pathol. 59, 437 (1970).

Lewis, J. H.: The antigenic relationship of alcohol-soluble fractions of brain and testicle. J. Immunol. 27, 473 (1934).

Lewis, R. M., Schwartz, R. S., Gilmore, C. E.: Autoimmune disease in domestic animals. Ann. N. Y. Acad. Sci. 124, 78 (1965).

Li, T., Behrman, S. J.: The sperm and seminal plasma specific antigens of human semen. Fertil. Steril. 21, 565 (1970).

Lippiello, L. A., El-Rubaye, F., Weil, A. J.: Human spermatozoa-coating antigen. Studies on purification. Fertil. Steril. 19, 991 (1968).

Lustig, L., Denduchis, B., Gonzalez, N., Mancini, R. E.: Chemical and immunologic study of rat seminiferous tubule wall structures. Acta physiol. lat.-amer. 23, 101 (1973).

Lustig, L., Denduchis, B., Gonzalez, N., Mancini, R. E.: Immuno-histochemical study of rat seminiferous tubule wall structures. Int. J. Fertil. 1976 (in press).

Mancini, R. E.: Allergic aspermatogenesis induced in man and animals. In: Injury, Inflammation and Immunity. p. 128 Thomas, L., Uhr, J. W., and Grant, L. (eds.), Baltimore: Williams & Wilkins, 1964.

Mancini, R. E.: Cellular and subcellular aspects of allergic orchitis. Proc. 1st. Symp. on Immunology and Reproduction. p. 49 Edwards, R. G. (Ed.), London: IPPF, 1968 a.

Mancini, R. E.: Experimental induction of antisperm antibodies with different testicular antigens in man. Proc. 6th. World Cong. on Fertil. Steril. Halbrecht, I. (Ed.), Tel Aviv: Israel Acad. Sciences and Humanities, 1968 b, p. 297.

Mancini, R. E.: Immunologic and testicular response to a damage induced in the contralateral gland. In: Male Fertility and Sterility. Mancini, R. E. and Martini, L. (eds.) New York: Academic Press 1974.

Mancini, R. E., Alonso, A., Gonzalez, N., Scacciati, J. M.: Bueno, M. P.: Antigenicity of guinea pig acrosomal fractions. Acta europ. Fertil. (1975) (in press).

Mancini, R. E., Alonso, A., Saraceni, A., Bachmann, A. E., Lavieri, J. C., Nemirovsky, M.: Immunological and testicular response in man sensitized with human testicular homogenate. J. clin. Endocr. 25, 859 (1965).

Mancini, R. E., Scacciati, J. M., Bueno, M. P.: Immunobiological properties of antisera against glycoproteins from human seminal plasma. Int. J. Fertil. (1976) (in press).

Mancini, R. E., Davidson, O. W., Vilar, O., Nemirovsky, M., Bueno, M. P.: Localization of acrosomal antigenicity in guinea pig testes. Proc. Soc. exp. Biol. Med. (N. Y.) 111, 435 (1962).

Mancini, R. E., Davidson, O. W., Vilar, O., Nemirovsky, M., Bueno, M. P.: Acrosomal antigenicity in rat testes. Fertil. Steril. 15, 695 (1964).

Mancini, R. E., Fainboim, L., Alonso, A.: Effect of homologous antisperm serum intratesticularly injected in guinea pigs. J. Allergy and Clin. Immunol. 54, 69 (1974).

Mancini, R. E., Gallo Morando, G., Torres Aguero, M., Pahul, G.: Homotransplantation of testis in dogs. I. Histologic study of the rejection phenomena. Medicina 32, 215 (1972).

Mancini, R. E., Gutierrez, O., Fernández Collazo, E.: Immunohistochemical localization of antigens in human spermatozoa. Fertil. Steril. 22, 475 (1971).

Mancini, R. E., Huidobro, H., Fernández Collazo, E., Monastirsky, R.: Detection of kininlike substances in the guinea pig testis after sensitization with homologous testicular extract. Proc. Soc. exp. Biol. Med. (N. Y.) 123, 227 (1966).

Mancini, R. E., Mazzolli, A., Thierer, E.: Immunological and testicular response of guinea pigs sensitized with homogenate from homologous thermal injured testis. Proc. Soc. exp. Biol. Med. 139, 991 (1972).

MANCINI, R. E., MONASTIRSKY, R., FERNÁNDEZ COLLAZO, E., SEIGUER, A. C., ALONSO, A.: Cytotoxic action of antispermatic antibodies upon homologous germinal cells "in vitro". Fertil. Steril. **20**, 779 (1969).

MANCINI, R. E., VILAR, O., ALVAREZ, B., SEIGUER, A. C.: Extravascular and intratubular diffusion of labeled serum proteins in the rat testis. J. Histochem. Cytochem. **13**, 376 (1965).

MARCUS, Z. H., SOFFER, Y., BEN-DAVID, A., PELEG, S., NEBEL, L.: Studies on sperm antigenicity. I. Delayed hypersensitivity to spermatozoa. European J. Immunol. **3**, 75 (1973).

MARUTA, H., MOYER, D. L.: Immunological studies of the antigens of guinea pig semen. Fertil. Steril. **18**, 649 (1967).

MATSUURA, H.: Immunological studies on spermatozoa. Japanese J. Exptl. Med. **26**, 75 (1956).

MATTILA, S.: Detection of two molecular forms of the human prostatic acid phosphatase. Invest. Urol. **6**, 337 (1969).

MAZZOLLI, A.: Demonstration "in vitro" of delayed hypersensitivity in experimental allergic orchitis in guinea pigs. J. Reprod. Fertil. **26**, 161 (1971).

MAZZOLLI, A., BARRERA, C.: A method for detecting cytophilic activity in a homologous system. J. Immunol. Method. **4**, 41 (1974).

MAZZOLLI, A., BUSTUOABAD, O., MANCINI, R. E.: Autologous sensitization to thermal orchitis homogenate. Immunological and testicular response. Int. J. Fert. (1976) (in press).

MENGE, A. C., PROTZMAN, W. P.: Origin of the antigens in rabbit semen which induce antifertility antibodies. J. Reprod. Fertil. **13**, 31 (1967).

METALNIKOFF, S.: Etudes sur la spermatoxine. Ann. Inst. Pasteur (Paris) **14**, 577 (1900).

METCHNIKOFF, E.: Recherches sur l'influence de l'organisme sur les toxines, sur le spermatoxine et l'antispermatoxine. Ann. Inst. Pasteur (Paris) **14**, 1 (1900).

MISCHLER, T. W., REINECKE, E. P.: Some electrophoretic and immunological properties of human semen. J. Reprod. Fertil. **12**, 125 (1966).

MITCHISON, N. A.: Induction of paralysis in two zones of dosage. Proc. Roy. Soc. London Ser. B **161**, 275 (1964).

MONCURE, C. W., PROUT, G. R., JR., BLAYLOCK, W. K.: Prostatic acid phosphatases antisera. Invest. Urol. **5**, 331 (1968).

MOXTER, D. VON: Über ein spezifisches Immunserum gegen Spermatozoen. Deutsche Med. Wchnschr. **26**, 21 (1900).

MOYER, D. L., MARUTA, H.: Induced isoantibody to homologous seminal and spermatozoal antigens in female monkeys. Fertil. Steril. **18**, 497 (1967).

MUDD, S., MUDD, E.: The specificity of mammalian spermatozoa with special reference to electrophoresis as a means of serological differentiation. J. Immunol. **17**, 39 (1929).

MUNFORD, D. M., BARSALES, P. B., BALE, K. D., GORDON, H. L.: Microlymphocyte transformation studies with seminal antigen. Technique and patterns of responsiveness to allogenic semen from normal and infertile male subjects. J. Urol. **105**, 858 (1971).

NAKABAYASHI, N. T., TYLER, E. T., TYLER, A.: Immunological aspects of human infertility. Fertil. Steril. **12**, 544 (1961).

NAKANE, P. K., PIERCE, G. B., JR.: Enzyme labeled antibodies for the light and electron microscopic localization of tissue antigens. J. Cell. Biol. **33**, 307 (1967).

NIESCHLAG, E., KLAUS-HENNING, U., SCHWEDES, U., KLEY, H. K., SCHÖFFLING, K., KRÜSKEMPER, H. L.: Alterations in testicular morphology and function in rabbits following active immunization with testosterone. Endocrinology **92**, 1142 (1973).

ORSINI, F., SHULMAN, S.: The antigens and autoantigens of the seminal vesicle. I. Immunochemical studies on guinea pig vesicular fluid. J. exp. Med. **134**, 120 (1971).

OTANI, Y., INO, H., KAGAMI, T.: Antigenicity of human semen, sperm and testis. Int. J. Fertil. **10**, 143 (1965).

PAGE, A. R., CONDIE, R. M., GOOD, R. A.: Suppression of plasma cell hepatitis with 6-mercapto-purine. Amer. J. Med. 36, 200 (1964).

PARISH, W. E., WARD, A.: Studies of the cervical mucus and serum from infertile women. J. Obstet. Gynaecol. Brit. Common. 75, 1089 (1968).

PATEL, S., SHULMAN, S.: Isolation of human sperm antigens. Fed. Proc. 33, 1 (1974).

PATERSON, P. Y., HARWIN, S. M.: Suppression of allergic encephalomyelitis by means of antibrain serum. J. exp. Med. 117, 755 (1963).

PECK, H. M., WOODHOUR, A. F., HILLEMAN, M. R.: New metabolizable immunologic adjuvant for human use. Chronic toxicity and teratogenic tests. Proc. Soc. exp. Biol. Med. 128, 699 (1968).

PEEL, S.: An immunologic study of dog prostate and the effects of injecting antidog prostate serum. Invest. Urol. 5, 427 (1968).

PERNOT, E., SZUMOWSKI, P.: Etude électrophorétique et immunoélectrophorétique des proteines du plasma séminal du taureau. Bull Soc. Chim. biol. 40, 1423 (1958).

PHADKE, A. M., PADUKONE, K.: Presence and significance of autoantibodies against spermatozoa in the blood of men with obstructed vas deferens. J. Reprod. Fertil. 7, 163 (1964).

PIKO, L.: Immunologic phenomena in the reproductive process. Int. J. Fertil. 12, 68 (1967).

POKORNÁ, Z.: Induction of experimental autoimmune aspermatogenesis by immune serum fractions. Folia. Biol. (Praha) 16, 320 (1970).

POKORNÁ, Z., VOJTISKOVÁ, M.: Ontogenic manifestation of the testicular antigen and the inducibility of autoimmune lesion by means of immature guinea pig testes. Folia Biol. (Praha) 10, 392 (1964 a).

POKORNÁ, Z., VOJTISKOVÁ, M.: Autoimmune damage of the testes induced with chemically modified organ specific antigen. Folia. Biol. (Praha) 10, 261 (1964 b).

POKORNÁ, Z., VOJTISKOVÁ, M.: Non-specific inhibition of various types of immune response by means of normal serum. Folia Biol. (Praha) 12, 88 (1966).

POKORNÁ, Z., VOJTISKOVÁ, M., RYCHLIKOVÁ, M., CHUTNÁ, J.: An isologous model of experimental autoimmune aspermatogenesis in mice. Folia Biol. (Praha) 9, 203 (1963).

POPIVANOV, R., STURKALEV, I., EVREV, T., NAKOV, L., ZHIVCOV, S., KIROV, K., RUSSEV, L., BOULANOV, I.: Proper and acquired blood group antigens in human testis cells and spermatozoa. p. 93 In.: Immunology of Spermatozoa and Fertilization. BRATANOV, K. (Ed.), Sofia: Bulgarian Academic Science Press 1969.

POPIVANOV, R., VULCHANOV, V. H.: Segregation of man's AB group spermatozoa in A and B spermatozoa through agglutination with immune anti-A rabbit serum. Z. Immun. Allergie-forsch. 124, 206 (1962).

QUIN, P. J., WHITE, S., CLELAND, K. W.: Chemical and ultrastructural changes in ram spermatozoa after washing, cold shock and freezing. J. Reprod. Fertil, 18, 209 (1969).

RAITSINA, S. S., NILOVSKY, M. N.: Post-traumatic aspermatogenesis. Resemblance of pathogenesis of autoallergic and post-traumatic orchitis. Folia Biol. (Praha) 13, 450 (1967).

RAO, S. S., SADRI, K. K.: Immunological studies with human semen and cervical mucus, p. 544. Proc. Sixth Internat. Conf. Planned Parenthood, New Delhi. The International Planned Parenthood Federation (Ed.), London: 1959.

RAO, S. S., SADRI, K. K.: The antigenic composition of buffalo semen. J. comp. Pathol. 70, 1 (1960).

RAO, S. S., SHETH, A. R.: Antigenicity of human spermatozoa and its significance, p. 1. In: Proc. Symp. on Proteins. Mysore, India. Central Food Technological Research Institute 1961.

RAPAPPORT, F. T., SAMPATH, A., KANO, K., MC CLUSKEY, R. T., MILGROM, F.: Immunological effects of thermal injury. I. Inhibition of spermatogenesis in guinea pigs. J. exp. Med. 130, 1411 (1969).

RICCI, M., ROMAGNANI, S., PASSALEVA, A., BILOTTI, G.: Lymphocyte transformation and macrophage migration in guinea pigs immunized with Freund's complete adjuvant. Clin. exp. Immunol. 5, 659 (1969).

RISLEY, P. L.: Physiology of the male accessory organs. In: Mechanism concerned with conception. HARTMAN, G. G. (Ed.), Oxford: Pergamon Press 1963.

ROBERTS, T. K., BOETTCHER, B.: Identification of human sperm-coating antigen. J. Reprod. Fertil. 18, 347 (1969).

ROTHBARD, S., WATSON, S. R.,: Amyloidosis and renal lesion induced in mice by injection with Freund-type of adjuvant. Proc. Soc. exp. Biol. Med. 85, 133 (1954).

RÜMKE, P.: The presence of sperm antibodies in the serum of two patients with extreme oligozoospermia. Vox. Sang. 4, 135 (1954).

RÜMKE, P.: Autospermagglutinins: A cause of infertility in men. Ann. N. Y. Acad. Sci. 124, 696 (1965).

RÜMKE, P.: Autoantibody formation against spermatozoa caused by extravasation of spermatozoa into the interstitium of the epididymis of aged men. Int. J. Fertil. 17, 86 (1972).

RÜMKE, P.: Antigens of semen and auto-immunitiy against spermatozoa in infertile men. In: Male Fertility and Sterility: MANCINI, R. E., and MARTINI, L. (eds.), New York: Academic Press 1974.

RÜMKE, P., HELLINGA, G.: Autoantibodies against spermatozoa in sterile men. Amer. J. clin. Pathol. 32, 357 (1959).

RÜMKE, P., TITUS, M.: Spermagglutinin formation in male rats by subcutaneously injected syngeneic epididymal spermatozoa and by vasoligation or vasectomy. J. Reprod. Fertil. 21, 69 (1970).

RÜMKE, P., VAN AMSTEL, M., MESSER, E. N., BEZEMER, P. D.: Prognosis of men with autospermagglutinins in the serum and the unsuccessful treatment with testosterone p. 339. Proc. IInd. Inter. Symp. on Immunology of Reproduction. BRATANOV, K., EDWARDS, R. G., VULCHANOV, V. H., DIKOV, V., SOMLEV, B. (eds.), Bulgarian Academy of Sciences Press 1973.

RUSSO, J., METZ, C. B.: The ultrastructural lesions induced by antibody and complement in rabbit spermatozoa. Biol. Reprod. 10, 293 (1974).

SADRI, K. K., SHETHYE, T. A., RAO, S. S.: Immunological and biological studies with antiserum to mouse testis extract. Indian J. exp. Biol. 5, 122 (1967).

SCACCIATI, J. M.: Studies on the trichloroacetic acid soluble fraction of the human seminal plasma. Anales Asoc. Quim. Argentina 59, 105 (1971).

SCACCIATI, J. M.: Physico-chemical studies of glycoproteins substances of human seminal plasma. Int. J. Fertil. 19, 211 (1975).

SCACCIATI, J. M., MANCINI, R. E.: Soluble and insoluble antigens of human spermatozoa. Fertil. Steril. 26, 1, 6 (1975).

SCHWARTZ, R. S., DAMESHEK, W.: Drug induced immunological tolerance. Nature 183, 1682 (1959).

SCHWIMMER, W. B., USTAY, K. A., BEHRMAN, S. J.: Spermagglutinating antibodies and decreased fertility in prostitutes. Obstet. Gynec. 20, 192 (1967 a).

SCHWIMMER, W. B., USTAY, K. A., BEHRMAN, S. J.: An evaluation of immunologic factors of infertility. Fertil. Steril. 18, 167 (1967 b).

SEARCY, R. L., CRAIG, R. G., BERGQUIST, L. M.: Immunochemical properties of normal and pathological seminal plasma. Fertil. Steril. 15, 1 (1964).

SHAW, C. M. FAHLBERG, W. J., KIES, M. W., ALVORD, C. E.: Suppression of experimental "allergic" encephalomyelitis in guinea pigs by encephalitogenic proteins extracted from homologous brain. J. exp. Med. 111, 171 (1960).

SHETHYE, T. A., RAO, S. S.: Aspermatogenesis induced by epididymal extract plus Freund's adjuvant in mice. Indian J. exp. Biol. 6, 123 (1968).

SHULMAN, S.: Antigenicity and autoimmunity in sexual reproduction: A review. Clin. Exp. Immunol. 9, 267 (1971).

SHULMAN, S.: Antibodies to spermatozoa. IV. Human spermagglutinating activity in different tests with variation in semen source. Fertil. Steril. (1974) (in press).

SHULMAN, S., AHMED, U.: Prostate antigens and antibodies. Proc. Soc. exp. Biol. (N. Y.) **137**, 97 (1971).

SHULMAN, S., BRONSON, P.: Immunochemical studies on human seminal plasma. II. The major antigens and their fractionation. J. Reprod. Fertil. **18**, 481 (1969).

SCHULMAN, S., FERBER, J.: Multiple forms of prostatic acid phosphatase. J. Reprod. Fertil. **11**, 295 (1966).

SHULMAN, S., HEKMAN, A.: Antibodies to spermatozoa. I. A new macroscopic agglutination technique for their detection. Clin. exp. Immunol. **9**, 137 (1971).

SHULMAN, S., HEKMAN, A., PANN, C.: Antibodies to spermatozoa. II. Spermagglutination techniques for guinea pigs and human cells. J. Reprod. Fertil. **27**, 31 (1971).

SHULMAN, S., ORSINI, F.: The antigens of seminal vesicles and seminal plasma. Fertil. Steril. **21**, 794 (1970).

SHULMAN, S., YANTORNO, C., BRONSON, P. M.: Cryoimmunology: a method of immunization to autologous tissue. Proc. Soc. exp. Biol. Med. **126**, 658 (1967).

SHULMAN, S., YANTORNO, C., SOANES, W. A., GONDER, M. J., WITEBSKY, E.: Studies on organ specificity. XVI. Urogenital tissues and autoantibodies. Immunolgy **10**, 99 (1966).

SOBBE, A., HAFERKAMP, O., DOEPFMER, R.: Serologische und immunohistologische Untersuchungen an Sperma und Seren von Männern steriler Ehen. Dtsch. med. Wschr. **91**, 1234 (1966).

SOLISH, G. I.: Distribution of ABO isohemagglutinins among fertile and infertile women. J. Reprod. Fertil. **18**, 459 (1969).

SOUTHAM, A. L.: Clinical significance of antibodies to spermatozoa and seminal plasma. J. Reprod. Fertil. **5**, 458 (1963).

SPOONER, R. L.: Cytolytic activity of the serum of normal male guinea pigs against their own testicular cells. Nature (Lond.) **202**, 915 (1964).

STEVENS, K. M., FOST, C. A.: Sperm and antibody formation in rabbits following immunization with sperm and semen. Proc. Soc. exp. Biol. Med. (N. Y.) **117**, 125 (1964).

STONE, S. H., LERNER, E. M., GOODE, J. H. (Jr.): Adoptive transfer of autoimmune aspermatogenesis in inbred guinea pigs p. 339. In.: International Convocation on Immunology. ROSE, N. R., and MILGROM, F. (eds), Basel: Karger 1969.

STRUBE, A.: Beiträge zum Nachweis von Blut und Eiweiß auf biologischem Weg. Dtsch. med. Wschr. **28**, 425 (1902).

SWANSON BECK, J., EDWARDS, R. G., YOUNG, M. R.: Immune fluorescence technique and the iso-antigenicity of mammalian spermatozoa. J. Reprod. Fertil. **4**, 103 (1962).

TOULLET, F., VOISIN, G. A.: Réactions d'hipersensibilité et anticorps serigues envers les auto-antigènes des spermatozoides. Relation avec le mécanisme de l'orchite aspermatogénétique auto-immune. Annls. Inst. Pasteur (Paris) **116**, 579 (1969).

TOULLET, F., VOISIN, G. A., NEMIROVSKY, M.: Immunohistochemical localization of the guinea pig spermatozoal autoantigens. Immunology **24**, 635 (1973).

TUNG, K. S. K., UNANUE, E. R., DIXON, F. J.: The immunopathology of experimental allergic orchitis. Amer. J. Pathol. **60**, 313 (1970).

TUNG, K. S. K., URANUE, E. R., DIXON, F. J.: Pathogenesis of experimental allergic orchitis. I. The role of antibody. J. Immunol. **6**, 1463 (1971 a).

TUNG, K. S. K., URANUE, E. R., DIXON, F. J.: Pathogenesis of experimental allergic orchitis. I. Transfer with lymph node cells. J. Immunol. **106**, 1453 (1971 b).

TYLER, A., TYLER, E. T., DENNY, P. C.: Concepts and experiments in immunoreproduction. Fertil. Steril. **18**, 153 (1967).

VESELSKY, L., MATOUSEK, J.: Auto- and isoimmunization of males with seminal plasma, p. 187. Proc. IInd. Inter. Symp. on Immunology of Reproduction. BRATANOV, K., EDWARDS, R. G., VULCHANOV, V. H., DIKOV, V., SOMLEV, B. (Eds.); Bulgarian Acad. of Science Press 1973.

VOISIN, G. A.: Immunity and tolerance: A unified concept. Cell. Immunol. **2**, 670 (1971).

VOISIN, G. A., DELAUNAY, A., BARBER, M.: Sur les lésions testicularies provoqueés chez le cobayes par iso- et autosensibilisation. Annls. Inst. Pasteuer (Paris) 81, 48 (1951).

VOISIN, G. A., TOULLET, F.: Etude sur l'orchite aspermatogenetique auto-immune et les autoantigénes des spermatozoides chez le cobaye. Annls. Inst. Pasteuer (Paris) 114, 727 (1968).

VOISIN, G. A., TOULLET, F.: Autoimmune aspermatogenic orchitis. A model for three possible mechanisms of autoimmune lesions. Folia Allergologica 18, 310 (1971).

VOISIN, G. A., TOULLET, F., MAURER, P.: The nature of tissular antigens with particular reference to autosensitization and transplantation immunity. Anm. N. Y. Acad. Sci. 73, 726 (1958).

VOJTISKOVÁ, M., POKORNÁ, Z.: Prevention of experimental allergic aspermatogenesis by thymectomy in adult mice. Lancet. 1964 I, 644.

VOJTISKOVÁ, M., POKORNÁ, Z.: Cellular antigens of mouse spermatozoa as possible markers of gene action. In.: Proc. Intern. Symp. on Genetics of the Spermatozoa, p. 160. BEATTY, R. A., and GLUECKSOHN-WAELSCH, S. (Eds.), Copenhagen: Bogtrykkeriet Forum 1971.

VOJTISKOVÁ, M., VIKLICKY, V., JIRSÁKOVÁ, A., NOUZA, K., POKORNÁ, Z.: Amethopterin treatment of experimental allergic aspermatogenesis in mice and morphological changes of lymphoid organs. Folia Biol. 11, 364 (1965).

VULCHANOV, V. H.: Testicular damage and autoantibody formation in guinea pigs immunized with homologous seminal vesicular fluid. p. 136. In.: Immunology and Reproduction. EDWARDS, R. G., International Planned Parenthood Federation, London (Ed.) 1969.

WAKSMAN, B. H.: A histologic study of the autoallergic testis lesion in the guinea pigs. J. exp. Med. 109, 311 (1959 a).

WAKSMAN, B. H.: Allergic encephalomyelitis in rats and rabbits pretreated with nervous tissue. J. Neuropathol. Exp. Neurol. 18, 397 (1959 b).

WEGELIN, C.: Über Spermiophagie im menschlichen Nebenhoden. Beitr. Path. Anat. 69, 281 (1921).

WEIL, A. J.: The spermatozoa coating antigen (SCA) of the seminal vesicle. Ann. N. Y. Acad. Sci. 124, 267 (1965).

WEIL, A. J., FINKLER, A. E.: Antigens of rabbit semen. Proc. Soc. exp. Biol. (N. Y.) 98, 794 (1958).

WEIL, A. J., LOTSEVALOV, O., WILSON, H.: Antigens of human seminal plasma. Proc. Soc. exp. Biol. Med. (N. Y.) 92, 606 (1956).

WEIL, A. J., RODENBURG, J. M.: The seminal vesicle as the source of the spermatozoa-coating antigen of the seminal plasma. Proc. Soc. exp. Biol. (N. Y.) 109, 567 (1962).

WELLERSON, R., WAGSTAFF, P., ASCULAI, F., HUDSON MARIE, KUPFERBERG, A. B.: Induction of a spermatogenesis in guinea pigs through immunization with lactate dehydrogenase-X-isozyme. Internat. J. Fertil. 19, 65 (1974).

WILSON, L.: Sperm agglutinins in human semen and blood. Proc. Soc. exp. Med. (N. Y.) 85, 652 (1954).

WILSON, J. T., JONES, N., KATSH, S.: Induction of aspermatogenesis by passive transfer of immune sera or cells. Int. Arch. Allergy 46, 172 (1972).

YANTORNO, C., DEBANNE, M. T., VOTTERO-CIMA, E.: Autoimmune orchitis induced by autoimmunization with seminal plasma in the rabbit. J. Reprod. Fertil. 27, 311 (1971).

YANTORNO, C., VIDES, M. A., VOTTERO-CIMA, E.: Studies on the macromolecular and antigenic composition of rabbit seminal plasma. J. Reprod. Fertil. 29, 229 (1972).

YANTORNO, C., VOTTERO-CIMA, E., GALMARINI, M.: Experimental autoimmune damage to rabbit male accessory glands. Invest. Urol. 10, 397 (1973).

ZAPPI, E., SHULMAN, S.: Early histological changes in experimental contralateral epididymo-orchitis in the rabbit. J. Reprod. Fertil. 36, 23 (1974).

ZETTERGREN, L.: Epididymitis spermostatica granulomatosa. Acta chir. scand. 114, 150 (1958).

Subject Index

Monographs
on Endocrinology

Editors: F. Gross, A. Labhart, M.B. Lipsett,
T. Mann, L.T. Samuls, J. Zander

H. ELIAS
Normal and Pathologic
Human Embryology:
Textbook and Atlas

With contributions by J.E. Pauly,
C.B. Severn
Distribution rights for Japan:
Igaku Shoin Ltd., Tokyo

Springer-Verlag
Berlin
Heidelberg
New York

Illustrated Human Embryology
Distribution rights for
U.K., Commonwealth, and the Traditional
British Market (excluding Canada):
Chapman & Hall Ltd., London
Distribution rights for Japan:
Igaku Shoin Ltd., Tokyo

Volume 1
H. TUCHMANN-DUPLESSIS,
G. DAVID, P. HAEGEL
Embryogenesis
Translator: L.S. Hurley

Volume 2
H. TUCHMANN-DUPLESSIS,
P. HAEGEL
Organogenesis
Translator: L.S. Hurley

Volume 3
H. TUCHMANN-DUPLESSIS,
M. AROUX, P. HAEGEL
Nervous System and Endocrine Glands
Translator: L.S. Hurley

A. LABHART
Clinical Endocrinology
Theory and Practice
With a Foreword by G.W. Thorn
In collaboration with numerous experts.
Translators: A. Trachsler, J. Dodsworth-
Phillips
Distribution rights for Japan:
Igaku Shoin Ltd., Tokyo

J. HAYWARD
Hormones and Human Breast Cancer
An Account of 15 Years Study
(Recent Results in Cancer Research,
Vol. 24)

**Invertebrate Endocrinology and
Hormonal Heterophylly**
Editor: W.J. Burdette

Springer-Verlag
Berlin
Heidelberg
New York